OKANAGAN COLLEGE LIBRARY

01365568

K

D0731520

RA 644 .A25 C75 1990
AIDS demographics
Crimp, Douglas
                            136556

AIDS DEMOGRAPHICS

DATE DUE

MAY 7 '92	APR 1 8 1996
OCT - 7 1992	APR - 7 1997
DEC - 7 1992	
FEB 1 8 1993	APR 2 5 1998
MAR - 4 1993	NOV - 8 1998
MAR 1 6 1993	MAR 3 0 2002
DEC 1 4 1993	APR 1 6 2002
MAR 2 8 1994	
AUG 1 0 1994	APR 3 0 2002
AUG 2 4 1994	
MAR 1 5 1995	
APR - 5 1995	
MAY - 3 1995	
NOV 2 9 1995	
JAN 1 6 1995	
JAN 1 6 1996	
APR - 2 1996	

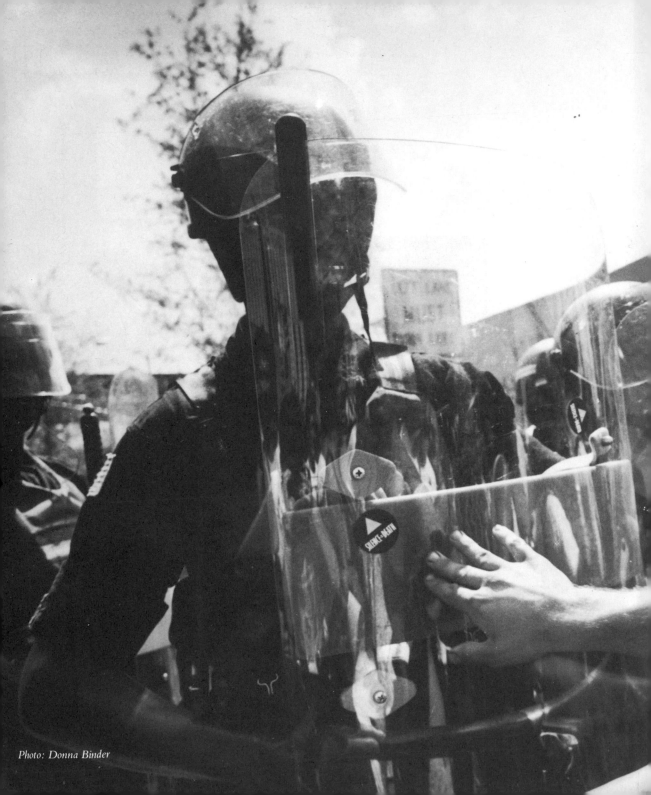

Photo: Donna Binder

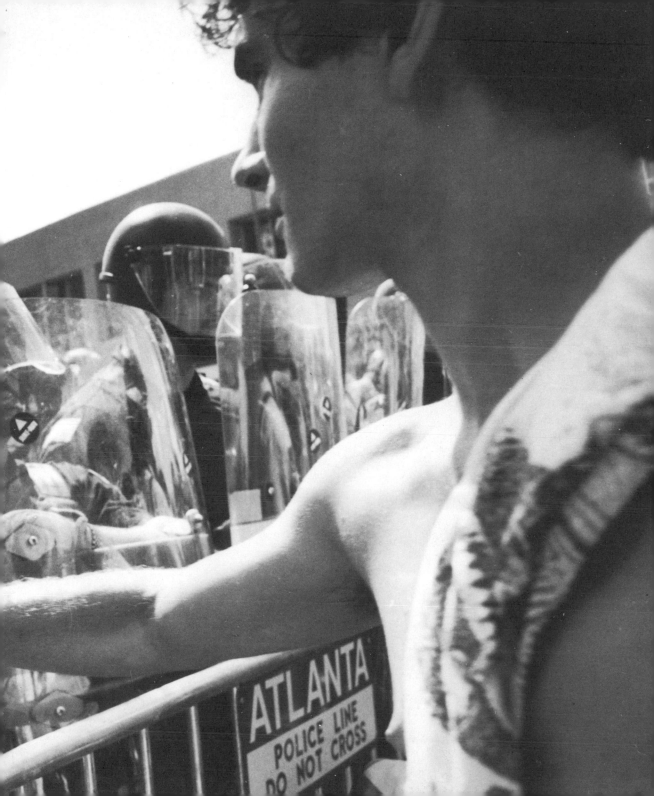

OKANAGAN COLLEGE LIBRARY
BRITISH COLUMBIA

AIDS DEMOGRAPHICS

Douglas Crimp
with Adam Rolston

Bay Press
Seattle
1990

© 1990 Douglas Crimp and Adam Rolston

All rights reserved. No part of this book may be reproduced in any form without permission in writing from the authors.

Printed in Korea

94 93 92 91   5 4 3 2

Bay Press

115 West Denny Way

Seattle, WA 98119

Design by Carin Berger

Production by Loch Adamson

Cover photo by Loring McAlpin from videotape by Catherine Saalfield

Typesetting by Trufont Typographers, Inc.

Set in Bembo and Futura

Library of Congress Cataloging-in-Publication Data

Crimp, Douglas.

AIDS demo graphics / Douglas Crimp with Adam Rolston.

        p.   cm.

Includes bibliographical references.

ISBN 0-941920-16-X (pbk.)

1. AIDS (Disease) – Political aspects.   2. AIDS (Disease) – Social aspects.   3. AIDS (Disease) – Posters.   I. Rolston, Adam, 1962–
II. Title.

RA644.A25C75   1990   89-81756

362.1'969792—dc20   CIP

This book is dedicated to the memory of the thousands who have died because of government inaction in the AIDS crisis, and to the survival of the millions who are fighting to stay alive.

13 | AIDS ACTIVIST GRAPHICS: A DEMONSTRATION

27 | NO MORE BUSINESS AS USUAL

29 | TAX DOLLARS FOR AIDS RESEARCH

32 | NATIONAL AIDS DEMO AT THE WHITE HOUSE

37 | ATEU AROUND-THE-CLOCK VIGIL

38 | DON'T GO TO BED WITH COSMO

43 | TRACKING THE PRESIDENTIAL COMMISSION

47 | WALL STREET II

53 | NINE DAYS OF PROTEST

72 | SURRENDER DOROTHY

76 | SEIZE CONTROL OF THE FDA

85 | TARGET CITY HALL

98 | STONEWALL 20

109 | ALL THE NEWS THAT'S FIT TO KILL

114 | SELL WELLCOME, FREE AZT

122 | HOUSING NOW

131 | STOP THE CHURCH

Like the graphics we illustrate, and like the ACT UP demonstrations we chronicle, this book is the product of collective effort. ACT UP's graphic artists and photographers donated their work and gave us detailed information. Various ACT UP members searched their files for the fact sheets—and their memories for the facts—that amplify the text. Material also came from ACT UP's publications, especially the collectively researched and compiled handbooks on the Food and Drug Administration, New York City AIDS issues, women and AIDS, AIDS and homelessness, and the history of the gay liberation movement. Gregg Bordowitz, Jean Carlomusto, D. A. Miller, and Donna Minkowitz—all ACT UP members—read the manuscript and provided useful comments. To everyone who helped, knowingly or unknowingly, we want to say thanks; thanks, too, to Thatcher Bailey of Bay Press for his enthusiastic support of this project, and to Carin Berger for the book's design.

—D.C. and A.R.

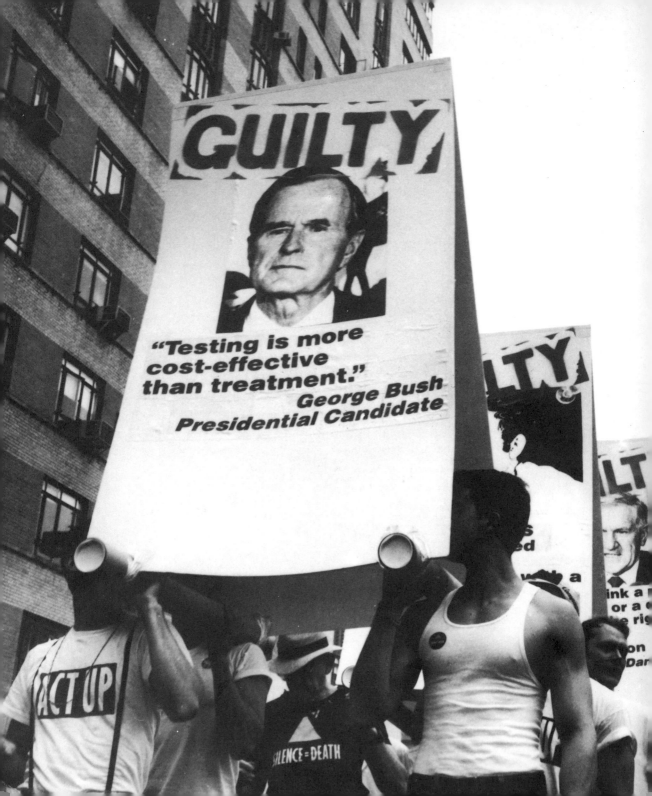

New York City, January 1990

This book is intended as a demonstration, in both senses of the word. It is meant as direct action, putting the power of representation in the hands of as many people as possible. And it is presented as a do-it-yourself manual, showing how to make propaganda work in the fight against AIDS. The AIDS activist graphics illustrated here were all produced by and for ACT UP, the AIDS Coalition to Unleash Power, "a diverse, nonpartisan group united in anger and committed to direct action to end the AIDS crisis." ACT UP New York was founded in March 1987. Subsequently, autonomous branches have sprung up in other cities, large and small, here and abroad–Chicago, Los Angeles, and San Francisco; Atlanta, Boston, and Denver; Portland and Seattle, Kansas City and New Orleans; Berlin, London, and Paris. Graphics are part of the action everywhere, but we confine ourselves to those associated with ACT UP New York as a matter of expediency. We live in New York–the city with the highest number of reported cases of AIDS in the world. We are members of ACT UP New York. We attend its meetings, join the debate, march in demonstrations, and get arrested for acts of civil disobedience here. And we're familiar with New York ACT UP's graphics, the people who make them, the issues they address. The limitation is part of the nature of our demonstration. We don't claim invention of the style or the techniques. We have no patent on the politics or the designs. There are AIDS activist graphics wherever there are AIDS activists. But ours are the ones we know and can show to others, presented in a context we understand. We want others to keep using our graphics and making their own. Part of our point is that nobody owns these images. They belong to a movement that is constantly growing–in numbers, in militancy, in political awareness.

Although our struggles are most often waged at the local level, the AIDS epidemic and the activist movement dedicated to ending it is national–and international–in scope, and the U.S. government is a major culprit in the problems we face and a central target of our anger. ACT NOW, the AIDS Coalition to Network, Organize, and Win–a national coalition of AIDS activist groups–has coordinated actions of national reach, most notably against the Food and Drug Administration (FDA) in October 1988. Health care is a national scandal in the United States; the FDA, the Centers for

Photo: Tom McKitterick

Disease Control (CDC), and the National Institutes of Health (NIH) are all critical to our surviving the epidemic, and we have monitored, lobbied, and fought them all. We have also taken our demands beyond U.S. borders. The Fifth International AIDS Conference in Montreal in June 1989 was *our* conference, the first of these annual, previously largely scientific and policy-making AIDS roundups to have its business-as-usual disrupted by the combative presence of an international coalition of AIDS activists. We took the stage–literally–during the opening ceremonies, and we never relinquished it. One measure of our success was that by the end of the conference perhaps one-third of the more than 12,000 people attending were wearing SILENCE = DEATH buttons.

That simple graphic emblem–SILENCE = DEATH printed in white Gill sanserif type underneath a pink triangle on a black ground–has come to signify AIDS activism to an entire community of people confronting the epidemic. This in itself tells us something about the styles and strategies of the movement's graphics. For SILENCE = DEATH does its work with a meta-phorical subtlety that is unique, among political symbols and slogans, to AIDS activism. Our emblem's significance depends on foreknowledge of the use of the pink triangle as the marker of gay men in Nazi concentration camps, its appropriation by the gay movement to remember a suppressed history of our oppression, and, now, an inversion of its positioning (men in the death camps wore triangles that pointed down; SILENCE = DEATH's points up). SILENCE = DEATH declares that silence about the oppression and annihilation of gay people, *then and now*, must be broken as a matter of our survival. As historically problematic as an analogy of AIDS and the death camps is, it is also deeply resonant for gay men and lesbians, especially insofar as the analogy is already mediated by the gay movement's adoption of the pink triangle.[1] But it is not merely what SILENCE = DEATH says, but also how it looks, that gives it its particular force. The power of this equation under a triangle is the compression of its connotation into a logo, a logo so striking that you ultimately *have* to ask, if you don't already know, "What does that mean?" And it is the answers we are constantly called upon to give to others–small, everyday direct actions–that make SILENCE = DEATH signify beyond a community of lesbian and gay cognoscenti.

Although identified with ACT UP, SILENCE = DEATH precedes the forma-tion of the activist group by several months. The emblem was created by six gay men calling themselves the Silence = Death Project, who printed the emblem on posters and had them "sniped" at their own expense.[2] The members of the Silence = Death Project were present at the formation of ACT UP, and they lent the organization their graphic design for placards used in its second demonstration—at New York City's main post office on April 15, 1987. Soon thereafter SILENCE = DEATH t-shirts, buttons, and stickers were produced, the sale of which was one of ACT UP's first means of fundraising.

Nearly a year after SILENCE = DEATH posters first appeared on the streets of lower Manhattan, the logo showed up there again, this time in a neon version as part of a window installation in the New Museum of Contemporary Art on lower Broadway. New Museum curator Bill Olander, a person with AIDS and member of ACT UP, had offered the organization the window space for a work about AIDS. An ad hoc committee was formed by artists, designers, and others with various skills, and within a few short months *Let the Record Show*, a powerful installation work, was produced. Expanding SILENCE = DEATH's analogy of AIDS and Nazi crimes through a photomural of the Nuremburg trials, *Let the Record Show* indicted a number of individuals for their persecutory, violent, homophobic statements about AIDS—statements cast in concrete for the installation—and, in the case of then president Ronald Reagan, for his six-year-long failure to make any statement at all about the nation's number-one health emergency. The installation also included a light-emitting diode (LED) sign programmed with ten minutes of running text about the government's abysmal failure to confront the crisis.[3] *Let the Record Show* demonstrated not only the ACT UP committee's wide knowledge of facts and figures detailing government inaction and mendacity, but also its sophistication about artistic techniques for distilling and presenting the information. If an art world audience might have detected the working methods of such artists as Hans Haacke and Jenny Holzer in ACT UP's installation, so much the better to get them to pay attention to it. And after taking in its messages, who would have worried that the work might be too aesthetically derivative, not original enough? The aesthetic values of the traditional art world are of little consequence to AIDS activists. What counts in activist art is its propaganda effect; stealing the procedures of other artists is part of the plan—if it works, we use it.

ACT UP's ad hoc New Museum art project committee regrouped after finishing *Let the Record Show* and resolved to continue as an autonomous collective—"a band of individuals united in anger and dedicated to exploiting the power of art to end the AIDS crisis." Calling themselves Gran Fury, after the Plymouth model used by the New York City police as undercover cars, they became, for a time, ACT UP's unofficial propaganda ministry and guerrilla graphic designers. Counterfeit money for ACT UP's first-anniversary demonstration, WALL STREET II; a series of broadsides for New York ACT UP's participation in ACT NOW's spring 1988 offensive, NINE DAYS OF PROTEST; placards to carry and T-shirts to wear to SEIZE CONTROL OF THE FDA; a militant *New York Crimes* to wrap around the *New York Times* for TARGET CITY HALL—these are some of the ways Gran Fury contributed to the distinctive style of ACT UP. Their brilliant use of word and image has also won Gran Fury a degree of acceptance in the art world, where they are now given funding for public artworks and invited to participate in museum exhibitions and to contribute "artist's pages" to *Artforum*.[4]

But, like the government's response to the AIDS activist agenda, the art world's embrace of AIDS activist art was long delayed.[5] Early in 1988, members of the three ACT UP groups Gran Fury, Little Elvis, and Wave Three protested at the Museum of Modern Art (MOMA) for its exclusion of AIDS activist graphics. The occasion was an exhibition organized by curator Deborah Wye called "Committed to Print: Social and Political Themes in Recent American Printed Art." Work in the show was divided into broad categories: gender, governments/leaders, race/culture, nuclear power/ecology, war/revolution, economics/class struggle/the American dream. The singleness of "gender" on this list, the failure to couple it with, say, "sexuality," already reveals the bias. Although spanning the period from the 1960s to the present, "Committed to Print" included no work about either gay liberation or the AIDS crisis. When asked by a critic at the *Village Voice* why there was nothing about AIDS, the curator blithely replied that she knew of no graphic work of artistic merit dealing with the epidemic. AIDS activists responded with a handout for museum visitors explaining the reasons for demonstrating:

- We are here to protest the blatant omission from "Committed to Print" of any mention of the lesbian and gay rights movement and of the AIDS crisis.

- By ignoring the epidemic, MOMA panders to the ignorance and indifference that prolong the suffering needlessly.

- By marginalizing 20 years of lesbian and gay rights struggles, MOMA makes invisible the most numerous victims of today's epidemic.

- Cultural blindness is the accomplice of societal indifference. We challenge the cultural workers at MOMA and the viewers of "Committed to Print" to take political activism off the museum walls and into the realm of everyday life.

The distance between downtown and uptown New York—and between its constituent art institutions—was rarely so sharply delineated as it was with MOMA's blindness to SILENCE = DEATH, for it was only a few months earlier that Bill Olander had decided to ask ACT UP to design *Let the Record Show*, after having seen the ubiquitous SILENCE = DEATH poster the previous year: "To me," he wrote, "it was among the most significant works of art that had been inspired and produced within the arms of the crisis."[6] For more traditional museum officials, however, a current crisis is perhaps less easy to recognize, since they "see" only what has become distant enough to take on the aura of universality. The concluding lines of MOMA curator Wye's catalogue essay betray this prejudice: "In the final analysis it is not the specific issues or events that stand out. What we come away with is a shared sense of the human condition: rather than feeling set apart, we feel connected."[7] The inability of others to "feel connected" to the tragedy of AIDS is, of course, the very reason we in the AIDS activist movement have had to fight—to fight even to be thought of as sharing in what those who ignore us nevertheless presume to universalize as "the human condition."

But there is perhaps a simpler explanation for MOMA's inability to see SILENCE = DEATH. The political graphics in "Committed to Print" were, it is true, addressed to the pressing issues of their time, but they were made by "bona fide" artists—Robert Rauschenberg and Frank Stella, Leon Golob and Nancy Spero, Hans Haacke and Barbara Kruger. A few collectives were included—Group Material and Collaborative Projects—and even a few ad hoc groups—Black Emergency Cultural Coalition and Artists and Writers Protest Against the War in Vietnam. But these were either well-established artists' organizations or groups that had been burnished by the passage of time, making the museum hospitable to them. The Silence = Death Project (whose AIDSGATE poster had been printed in the summer of 1987) and Gran Fury (who by the time of the MOMA show had completed their first poster, AIDS: 1 IN 61) were undoubtedly too rooted in movement politics for MOMA's curator to see their work within her constricted aesthetic perspective; they had, as yet, no artistic credentials that she knew of.

The distance between downtown and uptown is thus figured in more ways than one. For throughout the past decade postmodernist art has deliberately complicated the notion of "the artist" so tenaciously clung to by MOMA's curator. Questions of identity, authorship, and audience–and the ways in which all three are constructed through representation–have been central to postmodernist art, theory, and criticism. The significance of so-called appropriation art, in which the artist forgoes the claim to original creation by appropriating already-existing images and objects, has been to show that the "unique individual" is a kind of fiction, that our very selves are socially and historically determined through preexisting images, discourses, and events.

Young artists finding their place within the AIDS activist movement rather than the conventional art world have had reason to take these issues very seriously. Identity is understood by them to be, among other things, coercively imposed by perceived sexual orientation or HIV status; it is, at the same time, willfully taken on, in defiant declaration of affinity with the "others" of AIDS: queers, women, Blacks, Latinos, drug users, sex workers.[8] Moreover, authorship is collectively and discursively named: the Silence = Death Project, Gran Fury, Little Elvis, Testing the Limits (an AIDS activist video production group), DIVA TV (Damned Interfering Video Activist Television, a coalition of ACT UP video-makers), and LAPIT (Lesbian Activists Producing Interesting Television, a lesbian task group within DIVA). Authorship also constantly shifts: collectives' memberships and individual members' contributions vary from project to project.

Techniques of postmodernist appropriation are employed by these groups with a sly nod to art world precursors. In a number of early posters, for example, Gran Fury adopted Barbara Kruger's seductive graphic style, which was subsequently, and perhaps less knowingly, taken up by other ACT UP graphic producers. In the meantime, Gran Fury turned to other sources. Their best-known appropriation is undoubtedly the public service announcement on San Francisco (and later New York) city buses produced for "Art Against AIDS on the Road," under the auspices of the American Foundation for AIDS Research. Imitating the look of the United Colors of Benetton advertising campaign, Gran Fury photographed three stylish young interracial couples kissing and topped their images with the caption KISSING DOESN'T KILL: GREED AND INDIFFERENCE DO. The punch of the message, its implicit reference to the risk of HIV transmission, and its difference from a Benetton ad derive from a simple fact: of the three kissing couples, only one pairs boy with girl. If their sophisticated postmodern style has gained art world attention and much-needed funding for Gran Fury, the collective has accepted it only hesitantly, often biting the hand that feeds. Their first poster commission from an art institution was discharged with a message about art world complacency: WITH 42,000 DEAD, ART IS NOT ENOUGH. Familiar with the fate of most critical art practices—that is, with the art world's capacity to co-opt and neutralize them—Gran Fury has remained wary of their own success. Such success can ensure visibility, but visibility *to whom*?

For AIDS activist artists, rethinking the identity and role of the artist also entails new considerations of audience. Postmodernist art advanced a political critique of art institutions—and art itself as an institution—for the ways they constructed social relations through specific modes of address, representations of history, and obfuscations of power. The limits of this aesthetic critique, however, have been apparent in its own institutionalization: critical postmodernism has become a sanctioned, if still highly contested, art world product, the subject of standard exhibitions, catalogues, and reviews. The implicit promise of breaking out of the museum and marketplace to take on new issues and find new audiences has gone largely unfulfilled. AIDS activist art is one exception, and the difference is fairly easy to locate.

The constituency of much politically engaged art is the art world itself. Generally, artists ponder society from within the confines of their studios; there they apply their putatively unique visions to aesthetic analyses of social conditions. Mainstream artistic responses to the AIDS crisis often suffer from just such isolation, with the result that the art speaks only of the artist's private sense of rage, or loss, or helplessness. Such expressions are often genuine and moving, but their very hermeticism ensures that the audience that will find them so will be the traditional art audience.[9]

AIDS activist artists work from a very different base. The point of departure of the graphics presented in this book—and of the work in video mentioned here—is neither the studio nor the artist's private vision, but AIDS activism. Social conditions are viewed from the perspective of the movement working to change them. AIDS activist art is grounded in the accumulated knowledge and political analysis of the AIDS crisis produced collectively by the entire movement. The graphics not only reflect that knowledge, but actively contribute to its articulation as well. They codify concrete, specific issues of importance to the movement as a whole or to particular interests within it. They function as an organizing tool, by conveying, in compressed form, information and political positions to others affected by the epidemic, to onlookers at demonstrations, and to the dominant media. But their primary audience is the movement itself. AIDS activist graphics enunciate AIDS politics to and for all of us in the movement. They suggest slogans (SILENCE = DEATH becomes "We'll never be silent again"), target opponents (the *New York Times*, President Reagan, Cardinal O'Connor), define positions ("All people with AIDS are innocent"), propose actions ("Boycott Burroughs Wellcome"). Graphic designs are often devised in ACT UP committees and presented to the floor at the group's regular Monday night meetings for discussion and approval. Contested positions are debated, and sometimes proposed graphic ideas are altered or vetoed by the membership. In the end, when the final product is wheatpasted around the city, carried on protest placards, and worn on T-shirts, our politics, and our cohesion around those politics, become visible to us, and to those who will potentially join us. Sometimes our graphics signify *only* internally, as when an ACT UP affinity group went to TARGET CITY HALL wearing T-shirts silk-screened with a photograph of the actress Cher. The group adopted the movie star's name as a camp gesture, and each time someone asked what it meant, CHER became an acronym for whatever could be concocted on the spot: anything from "Commie Homos Engaged in Revolution" to "Cathy Has Extra Rollers."

ACT UP's humor is no joke. It has given us the courage to maintain our exuberant sense of life while every day coping with disease and death, and it has defended us against the pessimism endemic to other Left movements, from which we have otherwise taken so much. The adoption of the name CHER for an affinity group makes this point. A tradition of Left organizing, affinity groups are small associations of people within activist movements whose mutual trust and shared interests allow them to function autonomously and secretly, arrive at quick decisions by consensus, protect one another at demonstrations, and participate as units in coordinated acts of civil disobedience. ACT UP's affinity groups function in all of these ways, but our affinities, like our identities, are complexly constituted. Because being queer is an identity most of us share, one of our

Art Is Not Enough,
1988,
Gran Fury.
Poster, offset lithography,
18 × 13½".

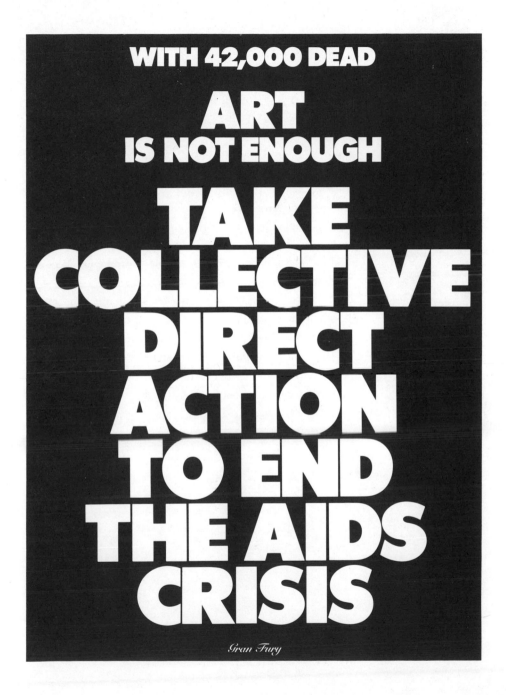

happiest affinities is camp. ACT UP graphics reflect that part of our politics too.

ACT UP has now become so adept at graphic production that we are able to have professionally produced posters even at "zaps," those small protests organized on the spur of the moment to respond to an emergency situation or a tip-off: the *New York Times* has just published a particularly damaging article; President Bush will be in town this week to speak at a Republican fundraiser; the New York City health commissioner is giving a lecture tomorrow at a health care facility. Having well-prepared visuals at such quickly arranged demonstrations is especially disarming to our opponents, who begin to fear our ubiquity. Protest movements have always had all-night poster-painting parties to prepare for such eventualities; ACT UP's innovation is to get the wheels of mechanical reproduction turning on equally short notice.

In addition to our large, well-organized demonstrations, ACT UP has staged hundreds of smaller protests and zaps over the past two and a half years. Most of them go unmentioned here, as do a few of our bigger demonstrations. The purpose of this book has been limited to presenting ACT UP's graphics in the context of demonstrations about major issues; we have therefore written only a partial history of a very complex political movement. One day in the future, when a far more complete history will be written, we hope ACT UP will have been just an episode–the episode compelled by the AIDS crisis–in the formation of a new mass movement for radical democratic change.

1. Although factions within the AIDS activist movement have employed holocaust metaphors indiscriminately–*genocide*, for example, is a term that often appears in early ACT UP fact sheets–it should be remembered that forced, punitive quarantine has been both a constant threat and, in some places and for some groups, a reality for people with HIV infection. For a detailed consideration of the gay and AIDS activist movements' adoption of the pink triangle, see Stuart Marshall, "The Contemporary Political Use of Gay History: The Third Reich," paper presented at *How Do I Look? A Queer Film and Video Conference*, Anthology Film Archives, New York, October 21–22, 1989 (conference papers forthcoming).

2. "Sniping" is a means of ensuring that posters pasted on hoardings will remain there for a specific time period without being covered over by anyone else's posters. In New York City, "snipers" are usually paid by promoters to put up rock concert advertisements and to replace them if they are torn down or pasted over.

3. For a more complete description of *Let the Record Show,* see the introduction to Douglas Crimp, ed., *AIDS*: *Cultural Analysis/Cultural Activism* (Cambridge, Massachusetts: MIT Press, 1988), pp. 7–12.

4. Gran Fury, "Control," *Artforum* 28 (October 1989), pp. 129–30, 167–68.

5. Long, that is, in relation to how time is and must be figured in the AIDS crisis. We do not mean to imply that the agenda of AIDS activist artists includes any special interest in art world acceptance–far from it. The art world is only one of many sites of struggle. Our point is that, whatever the position of AIDS activist artists, art institutions should recognize all vital forms of aesthetic production.

6. Bill Olander, "The Window on Broadway by ACT UP," in *On View* [handout] (New York: New Museum of Contemporary Art, 1987), p. 1.

7. Deborah Wye, *Committed to Print: Social and Political Themes in Recent American Printed Art* (New York: Museum of Modern Art, 1988), p. 10.

8. "I am a member of the gay community and a member of the AIDS community. Furthermore, I am a gay member of the AIDS community, a community that some would establish by force, for no other end but containment, toward no other end but repression, with no other end but our deaths–a community that must, instead, establish *itself* in the face of this containment and repression.

We must proudly identify ourselves as a coalition" (Gregg Bordowitz, writing about the Testing the Limits video collective, in "Picture a Coalition," *AIDS: Cultural Analysis/Cultural Activism*, p. 195).

9. Individual artists' aesthetic responses to AIDS have not always been genuine or moving; sometimes they are exploitative and damaging. To take a notorious example, Nicholas Nixon's serial photographic portraits of people with AIDS (PWAs) reinforce mainstream media stereotypes of PWAs as isolated, despairing victims. When the photographs were shown at the Museum of Modern Art in the fall of 1988, ACT UP members protested, demanding NO MORE PICTURES WITHOUT CONTEXT. Part of the context excluded from Nixon's pictures, of course, is everything that kills people with AIDS besides a virus—everything that AIDS activists, PWAs among us, are fighting.

Photo: T. L. Litt

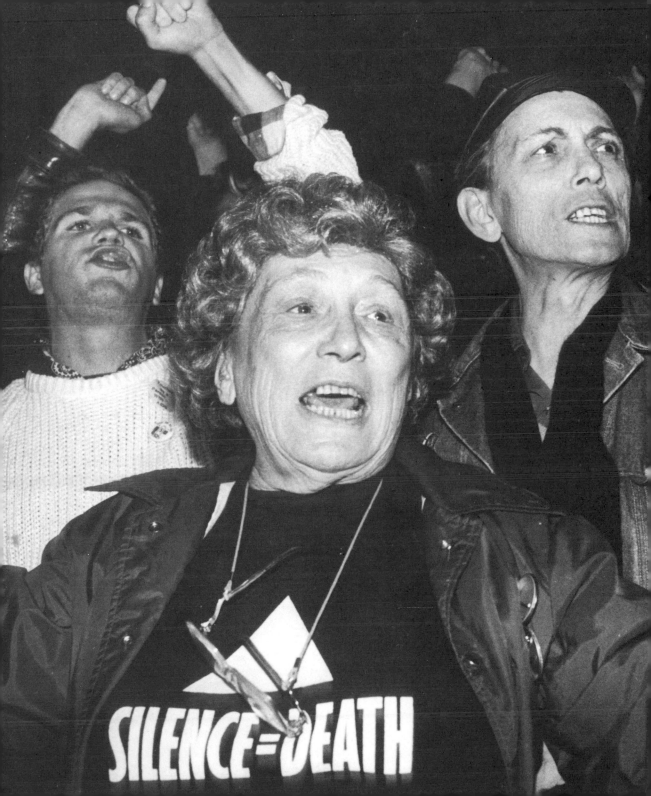
SILENCE=DEATH

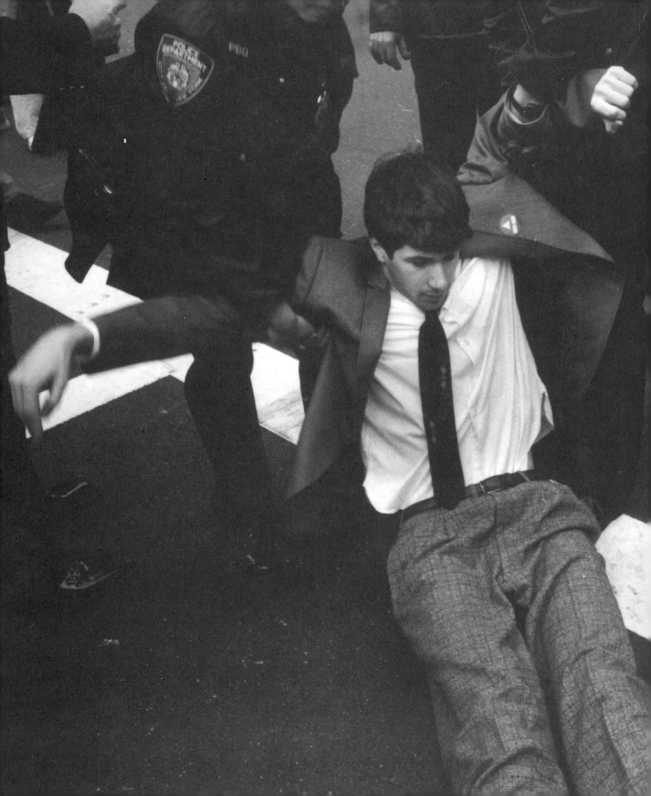

Wall Street, New York City, March 24, 1987

On March 10, 1987, Larry Kramer agreed to replace Nora Ephron in a monthly speaker's series at New York's Lesbian and Gay Community Services Center. As a founder of the Gay Men's Health Crisis, the author of *The Normal Heart*, and the most vocal critic of both official and community apathy about the AIDS epidemic, Kramer drew a large crowd of mostly gay men–the curious, the frightened, and the furious. Kramer began by citing his first call to action, "1,112 and Counting," published four years earlier in the *New York Native*. "Our continued existence," he had written, "depends on just how angry you can get." Now the situation was even more urgent: at the time of the community center speech, officially reported cases of AIDS in the United States had reached 32,000. Kramer produced a number of incitements to the mounting anger: a collapsing New York City health care system, an insurance industry that won't reimburse for home health care or experimental drugs, government officials who can't be bothered. But Kramer's main concern was the unavailability of treatments for AIDS owing to the Food and Drug Administration's snail-paced approval process. He condemned both the National Institutes of Health and the Food and Drug Administration for their inhumane and bureaucratic procedures, and he named a few promising drugs–ampligen, ribavirin, AL-721–on which the FDA refused to act. The exception was AZT (azidothymidine), highly toxic and highly profitable for its maker, Burroughs Wellcome.

Kramer then turned his criticism to New York's leading AIDS service organization, the Gay Men's Health Crisis (GMHC). Six weeks before, he had castigated the organization for a failure of nerve, and now he reiterated his demands: "lobbying, an advocacy division, more public-relations people to get the word out, a change of its tax-exempt status to allow for increased political activities, fighting for drugs. . . ." Discouraged by GMHC's inability to act politically given its corporate structure and service orientation, Kramer posed what turned out to be the crucial question to his audience: "Do we want to start a new organization devoted solely to political action?"

The answer was a resounding yes. Discussion following Kramer's speech ended in the resolve to meet again two days later, a meeting at which nearly 300 people would form the AIDS Coalition to Unleash Power.

Photo: Tom McKitterick

ACT UP, "a diverse, nonpartisan group united in anger and committed to direct action to end the AIDS crisis," set about immediately to plan its first demonstration, to take place March 24 on Wall Street. The target: BUSINESS, BIG BUSINESS, BUSINESS AS USUAL.

Licensing of the antiviral drug AZT, the only government-sanctioned new therapy for AIDS, was announced by the FDA on March 19. The exceptional rush through the FDA's bureaucratic approval process looked suspicious, since the agency was far from willing to do this for any other drug (AZT took just over two years to approve, as compared to the usual eight to ten). Burroughs Wellcome, the pharmaceutical company granted the monopoly, announced that it would charge each patient upwards of $10,000 annually, making AZT the costliest drug ever.

Over 250 ACT UP novices descended on Wall Street at 7 A.M. on a Thursday to protest the alliance between the FDA and Burroughs Wellcome in the interest of profit rather than saving lives. An effigy of FDA commissioner Frank Young was hung in front of Trinity Church. Traffic was tied up for several hours, and 17 people were arrested for acts of civil disobedience.

Larry Kramer had published an op-ed piece in the *New York Times* the previous day; in it he outlined the same grievances against the FDA that he had presented in his speech at the community center two weeks earlier. Thousands of copies were reproduced and handed out to crowds on their way to work in the financial district. ACT UP also produced its own fact sheet, asserting AIDS IS EVERYBODY'S BUSINESS NOW. The following points explained WHY WE ARE ANGRY:

- For 12 long months AZT was proclaimed as promising but in such short supply that it had to be rationed to a very few mortally ill patients. Once Burroughs Wellcome was licensed to distribute AZT, supply for **30,000** was immediately on hand!

- The National Institutes of Health continue inhumane double-blind placebo-controlled studies on terminal patients, but make no plans to experiment on the hundreds of thousands with AIDS-related complex (ARC) or HIV infection.

- Every major insurance company routinely denies benefits to people with AIDS or at risk for AIDS. That leaves only taxpayer-funded Medicaid, which will not pay for any form of experimental therapy.

- Even the surgeon general says the president must somehow be embarrassed into taking action. **Six years** into the worst pandemic in modern history, there are still no public education programs for everyone—not from the city, not from the state, not from the schools, not from the churches, not from the media.

- **Who is in charge?** The chief executive of this nation has yet to utter the word AIDS.

The demonstration and arrests made national news, and several weeks later, when Commissioner Young announced a speedup of the FDA's drug approval process, CBS anchor Dan Rather credited ACT UP's pressure.

TAX DOLLARS FOR AIDS RESEARCH

General Post Office, New York City, April 15, 1987

ACT UP's second demonstration was organized for the night of April 15 on the steps of New York City's main post office at Eighth Avenue and 33rd Street. Because the General Post Office stays open around the clock, hundreds of taxpayers go there to file their returns before the midnight deadline—thus becoming a captive audience for a demonstration about how much of their tax money would be spent to fight AIDS. Captive, also,

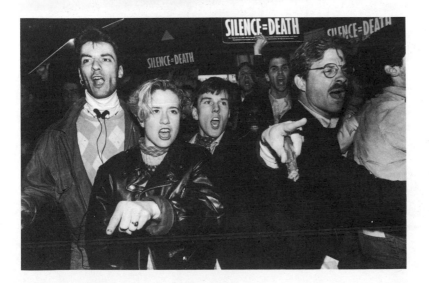

ACT UP demonstration at the General Post Office, New York City, April 15, 1987 (photo: Donna Binder).

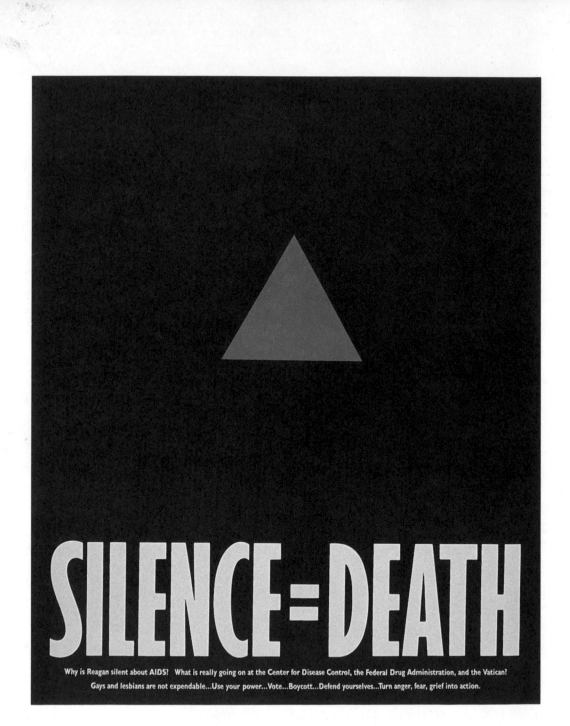

would be the electronic media, who routinely do stories about down-to-the-wire tax-return filers. ACT UP's media savvy thus showed itself from the very beginning, as did our ability to influence coverage by visual means. The Silence = Death Project members, who had printed their posters and wheatpasted them around Manhattan several months earlier, now mounted scores of them on foamcore to make placards for the taxpayer demo. When TV newscasters went to the post office that night, they returned with a new graphic image of ACT UP in action—one that would become increasingly identified with ACT UP as time went on. They also returned with a press release with our demands:

- **Immediate** establishment of a coordinated, comprehensive, and compassionate national policy on AIDS.

- **Immediate** release of drugs that may help save our lives.

- **Immediate** establishment of a $60 million fund to pay for AZT and other drugs as they become available.

- **Immediate** mass national education.

- **Immediate** policy to prohibit discrimination.

The taxpayers, too, were given something to take home—a letter addressed to President Reagan, which said, in part:

> Dear Mr. President:
> As a taxpayer and concerned citizen, I am writing to receive answers to some very pressing questions on your administration's handling of the AIDS epidemic.
>
> Why have the Centers for Disease Control failed to mount a national AIDS-prevention education campaign, even though $70 million was allocated for that purpose this year?
>
> Why is Burroughs Wellcome permitted to charge its asking price of $10,000 annually for AZT when the drug was developed with the help of government funds?
>
> Why haven't you, Mr. President, read your own surgeon general's report on AIDS, which was prepared in October 1986? Since then, over 4,800 Americans have died from this disease.

Silence = Death,
1986,
Silence = Death Project.
Poster, offset lithography,
29 × 24"
(also used as placard,
T-shirt, button, and
sticker).

In all, your administration has witnessed almost 20,000 deaths from AIDS. When will you see fit to have your **f i r s t** meeting with the surgeon general to discuss the epidemic?

HOW MUCH LONGER MUST WE WAIT??

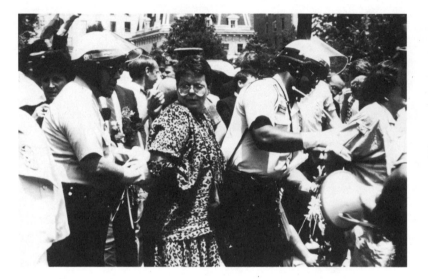

Police arrest AIDS activists at the White House, Washington, D.C., June 1, 1987 (photo: Jane Rosett).

N A T I O N A L   A I D S   D E M O   A T   T H E   W H I T E   H O U S E

Washington, D.C., June 1, 1987

The Third International Conference on AIDS was scheduled to open in Washington, D.C., on June 1, 1987, and activist groups from around the country descended on the capital to protest the Reagan administration's do-nothing record. The White House resident did his part to ensure the demonstration's media success when he addressed the opening ceremonies of the conference the evening of May 31. Speaking the word *AIDS* publicly for the first time since the beginning of the epidemic six years earlier, Reagan's only proposal was to demand widespread routine testing, for which he was loudly booed—not the president's usual reception from doctors, scientists, public health officials, and fundraisers like Liz Taylor, and a sure media story. Reagan's unwelcome call for testing was seconded by then vice president George Bush, speaking at the conference on the following evening; the booing was repeated. Bush, thinking the microphone wouldn't pick up his words, leaned over to an aide and asked, "What is it, some kind of gay group out there?"

But the most visible gaffe was produced by the Washington police. In front of the White House, cops wore bright-yellow rubber gloves as they arrested 64 protesters, thus fueling America's already fever-pitch hysteria about "catching" AIDS through casual contact. The activists, many looking unusually respectable in conservative business clothes, raised the very queer chant

YOUR GLOVES DON'T MATCH YOUR SHOES!
YOU'LL SEE IT ON THE NEWS!

The issue, though, was deadly serious. Just one year earlier, Reagan's attorney general, the not-quite-provable criminal Edwin Meese, ruled that a person with AIDS, or anyone suspected of having AIDS, could be fired so long as the employer claimed ignorance of the medical fact, quoted in the ruling itself, that there is no known health danger from workplace contact. And of course the employer's ignorance could be virtually guaranteed, since the federal government had not yet undertaken a national AIDS education campaign. Nor had it within the ensuing year. ACT UP therefore demanded, on a flier handed out at the White House, both a national education campaign and legislation to prohibit discrimination in employment, housing, insurance, and health care. Also included on the flier were two of the most alarming statistics ACT UP had learned:

- In **o n e   d a y** the Pentagon spends more than the **t o t a l** spent for AIDS research and education since 1982.

- By 1991, more Americans will die from AIDS **e a c h   y e a r** than were killed in the **e n t i r e** Vietnam war.

The national scandal of the Reagan administration's inaction on AIDS became the subject of the Silence = Death Project's second poster image, produced for the White House demonstration. It was the summer of congressional hearings about secret diversions to the Nicaraguan contras of funds from illegal arms sales to Iran–a series of events variously referred to as Irangate or Contragate, the "-gate" of Watergate having become the colloquial suffix for scandal. For their new graphic, the Silence = Death Project attached the scandal suffix to AIDS and stamped a shocking-pink

AIDSGATE over a Warhol-like picture of Reagan's ugly mug–made a little uglier with the repetition of the hot pink in the whites of the president's eyes. A caption at the bottom stated THIS POLITICAL SCANDAL MUST BE INVESTIGATED!

For nearly a year following the White House demonstration, the SILENCE = DEATH and AIDSGATE graphics were the main images at ACT UP's actions. Supplementary posters geared to specific issues were quickly improvised at poster parties prior to particular events, but it was the two Silence = Death Project works that gave ACT UP its well-organized, professional look–all the more so when we wore the two images on T-shirts as well. This look was itself a kind of organizing tool. ACT UP started out fairly small and has always been entirely open, leaderless, grass-roots, anarcho-democratic. But the impressive appearance of the group made people on the sidelines curious: something's happening here; I want to know what it is.

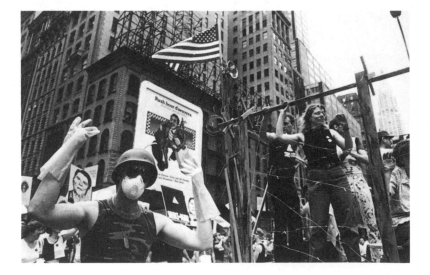

ACT UP "quarantine camp" in the gay pride march, New York City, June 28, 1987 (photo: Donna Binder).

ACT UP was a singular presence in New York's 1987 annual gay pride march during the last weekend in June. A float trimmed with barbed wire and driven by a man in a Ronald Reagan mask represented an AIDS quarantine camp. Surrounding it on the street were internment camp guards wearing gas masks and the now infamous yellow rubber gloves. Scores of activists followed with SILENCE = DEATH and AIDSGATE placards,

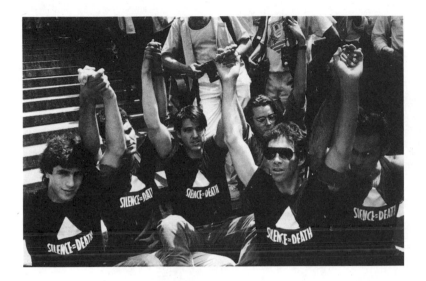

ACT UP demonstration at Federal Plaza, New York City, June 30, 1987 (photo: Donna Binder).

while others handed out leaflets announcing a rally and demonstration at the Jacob K. Javits Federal Building in lower Manhattan for the following week. Twice as many people were arrested at Federal Plaza for civil disobedience as in ACT UP's first demonstration on Wall Street just a few months before. A handout about THE GOVERNMENT'S **REAL** POLICY ON AIDS gave some of our reasons for risking arrest:

- The Social Security Administration has recently begun denying benefits to persons with AIDS because *"They may be dying, but they might not be disabled."*

- Almost every state is now considering testing or quarantine legislation. Senator Jesse Helms, who sponsored the alien testing bill in Washington, has declared *"The logical outcome of testing is a quarantine of those infected."*

- In 1988, mandatory testing of aliens and Veterans' Administration hospital patients alone will cost over $240 million, *more than Reagan's entire budget for drug research and vaccine development.*

Perhaps ACT UP's most impressive early appearance was at the massive March on Washington for Lesbian and Gay Rights, Columbus Day weekend, October 1987. AIDS was on nearly everyone's mind that weekend, not only because of the devastation of our communities, but also because of the initial unveiling of the Names Project quilt at dawn before the march. The quilt has grown horrifyingly larger since then—when it occupied the mere

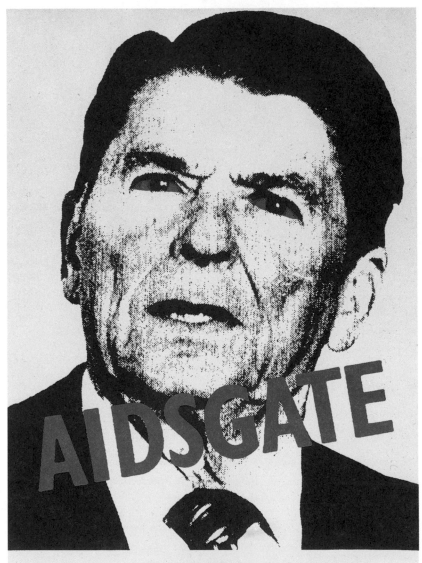

AIDSGATE

This Political Scandal Must Be Investigated!

54% of people with AIDS in NYC are Black or Hispanic... AIDS is the No. 1 killer of women between the ages of 24 and 29 in NYC...
By 1991, more people will have died of AIDS than in the *entire* Vietnam War... What is Reagan's *real* policy on AIDS?
Genocide of all Non-whites, Non-males, and Non-heterosexuals?...
SILENCE = DEATH

space of two football fields on the mall—but because no one had seen it before, it stunned the half million of us at the march.

Leading the 500,000 march participants were people with AIDS, some in wheelchairs pushed by their friends—a reminder that fighting AIDS is now a priority for gay people and that first in the fight are people living with AIDS. ACT UP was positioned toward the back of the march, our legions immediately recognizable from our SILENCE = DEATH T-shirts. SILENCE = DEATH and AIDSGATE posters had been mounted recto-verso on foamcore and hinged together to make a long serpentine of repeated graphic images, like a Chinese new-year dragon adapted for political action. If you were wearing one of our T-shirts, you could be sure to be asked countless times, "Who is that group?" On the following Monday night in New York, the weekly ACT UP meeting swelled to double its usual number—a sure sign that graphics are an aid to organizing.

ATEU AROUND-THE-CLOCK VIGIL

Memorial Sloan-Kettering Hospital, New York City, July 21–24, 1987

For the first six months or more of its existence, ACT UP had one dominant focus: "drugs into bodies." No matter what the occasion or site of a demonstration—Wall Street, the post office, the White House, Federal Plaza—the central issue was getting AIDS treatments out of the NIH and FDA bureaucracies and into the bodies of those who are HIV-infected. Inequalities in access to health care based on class, race, sex, and sexuality; AIDS-related discrimination in housing, jobs, and public accommodations; lack of explicit, culturally sensitive risk-reduction education; the disproportionately high number of people of color with AIDS; the special problems of prisoners, sex workers, drug users, and pregnant women—all these issues were discussed in meetings and mentioned on fact sheets, but the bottom line was treatment.

Treatment issues are extremely complicated and difficult to convey to an uninformed public. But groups within ACT UP began studying the situation intensively at a very early stage. Within the Issues Committee (since split into separate committees for various issues), there were initially two subcommittees working on treatment, one devoted to tracking treatment information generally, another concentrating on the system of AIDS

AIDSgate,
1987,
Silence = Death Project.
Poster, offset lithography,
34 × 22"
(also used as placard and
T-shirt).

Treatment Evaluation Units (ATEUs) established and funded by the NIH to test new AIDS therapies. In June 1986, Congress appropriated $47 million for the ATEU system of 19 medical centers across the country, where 12,000 people with AIDS were to be enrolled in drug trials. In the summer of 1987, ACT UP learned that after one year only 844 people had been enrolled, and that of these, 92 percent were in ongoing trials for AZT, already approved by the FDA several months before. Meanwhile, our Treatment and Data Subcommittee had researched a whole list of drugs showing promise for the treatment of AIDS that were not being tested. ACT UP decided to target one of the four ATEUs in New York City for a demonstration that would both apply pressure for increased clinical trial enrollment and educate the public about the dysfunctional ATEU system.

Between July 21 and 24, ACT UP staged an around-the-clock vigil at Memorial Sloan-Kettering Hospital, a designated ATEU with $1.2 million of funding from the NIH and a trial enrollment of only 31 patients. A fact sheet cogently outlined the situation, provided statistics detailing under-enrollment, and listed promising drugs not being tested. The response of the Sloan-Kettering medical staff was so positive that ACT UP issued a flier thanking them and providing information about how they could help, including writing to members of congressional committees dealing with health issues. Within the year, Manhattan congressman Theodore Weiss initiated a series of investigations. During one of these, Anthony Fauci, head of the National Institute of Allergy and Infectious Diseases, was forced to admit under oath that the ATEU system was not working, in part owing to staff shortages that he had remained silent about for over a year.

DON'T GO TO BED WITH COSMO

Hearst Magazine Building, New York City, January 19, 1988

In its January 1988 issue, *Cosmopolitan* magazine published "Reassuring News about AIDS: A Doctor Tells Why *You* May Not Be at Risk." The doctor in question was Robert E. Gould, a psychiatrist whose "concern" about AIDS was how to answer his women patients' growing fears of infection. His comforting answer: straight women have little to worry about, even if their sex partners are infected, and condom use is unneces-sary unless there are vaginal lacerations. Gould's lethal advice was based

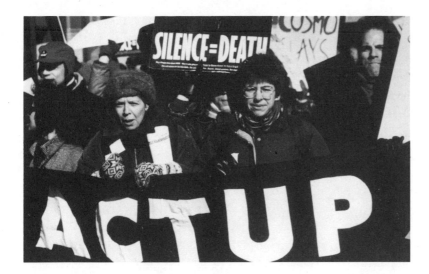

ACT UP says no to Cosmo *at the Hearst Magazine Building, New York City, January 19, 1988 (photo: Gerri Wells).*

entirely on ignorance and prejudice. It ignored recent statistics showing growing numbers of women infected through heterosexual intercourse; it accused women of lying about their sex lives, claiming, for example, that women won't "admit" to engaging in anal intercourse; and it "explained" the high incidence of heterosexually transmitted HIV infection in Africa with racist presumptions about differing sexual practices (for example, "Many men in Africa take their women in a brutal way, so that some heterosexual activity regarded as normal by them would be closer to rape by our standards."). *Cosmopolitan's* readership consists of women from ages 18 to 34–15 million of them worldwide; in New York City, AIDS is the leading cause of death in women aged 25 to 34. In January 1988, the Centers for Disease Control reported nearly 2,000 cases of AIDS among women, 26 percent of whom had no risk factor other than unprotected heterosexual intercourse with an infected partner.

By the time of the publication of the *Cosmo* article, a group of ACT UP women had been getting together at informal "dyke dinners" for several months to discuss the role of women, *lesbian* women in particular, in AIDS activism. That role often took the form in Monday night meetings of broadening the debate, keeping inequities determined by class, race, and sex on the agenda. But with the *Cosmo* article, the women had a galvaniz-ing issue specific to the lives of women, and they quickly swung into action to form a Women's Committee and organize a demonstration. On a wintry cold Tuesday nearly 150 activists crowded in front of the Hearst

Magazine Building on West 57th Street, where *Cosmopolitan* has its offices. Shouting SAY NO TO COSMO and handing out condoms and fliers to the lunchtime crowds, ACT UP alerted women to the danger *Cosmo* was putting them in and called for a boycott of the magazine and its advertisers (a list of advertisers' addresses was distributed).

The story was taken up—and taken away from the ACT UP women—by the national media. Women activists, who had accumulated extensive knowledge about women and AIDS, were physically ejected from a local talk show, *People Are Talking*, when they protested that the issues were being represented only by men. These same women found themselves blacklisted when they attempted to get into the studio audience of the *Phil Donahue Show* where Gould was appearing as a guest. And only an officially sanctioned expert, Dr. Mathilde Krim, founding chairperson of the American Foundation for AIDS Research, appeared against *Cosmo* editor Helen Gurley Brown and Dr. Gould on ABC's *Nightline*. But the ACT UP women did not simply stand back and watch the representation of their concerns be stolen from them. Members of the ACT UP Women's Committee who had organized the *Cosmo* demo quickly produced the highly praised documentary *Doctors, Liars, and Women: AIDS Activists Say No to Cosmo*. Aired on the Gay Men's Health Crisis weekly cable program *Living with AIDS* and widely circulated at video festivals, universities, museums, and community centers, the video not only presents a counterargument to *Cosmo*'s lies (Gould was naive enough to allow the videotaping of his meeting with ACT UP women), but also provides information on how to organize a demonstration and on the role of women in AIDS activism, including the role of self-representation.

In an open letter to *Cosmo*, Dr. Krim wrote, "The '*You*' to whom Dr. Gould addresses his article are obviously not—in his mind—any of those young minority-group women who give birth to HIV-antibody-positive babies at the rate, now, of **1 out of every 61** births occurring in New York City." That alarming statistic had recently been widely publicized, and, concurrently with the action organized by the ACT UP Women's Committee, Gran Fury produced their first poster, AIDS: 1 IN 61. The poster publicized not only the growing incidence of pediatric AIDS cases, but also the obvious—but apparently not to everyone—concurrent incidence of AIDS in those babies' mothers.

The *Cosmo* article was just one of many media stories that sought to

The AIDS Crisis Is Not Over,
1988,
Little Elvis.
Crack-and-peel sticker,
offset lithography,
3⅛ × 11" (also 1⅝ × 5½").

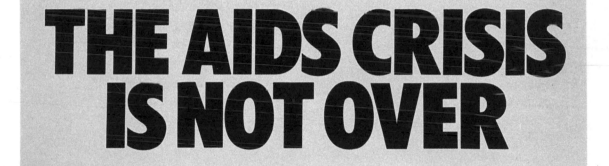

AIDS: 1 in 61

One in every sixty-one babies
in New York City is born with AIDS
or born HIV antibody positive.

So why is the media telling us
that heterosexuals aren't at risk?

Because these babies are black.
These babies are Hispanic.

Ignoring color ignores the facts of AIDS.
STOP RACISM: FIGHT AIDS.

Uno de cada sesenta y uno de los bebés nacidos
en la ciudad de New York nacen con SIDA,
o con el anticuerpo HIV positivo.

¿Pero, por qué es que los medios de comunicación
nos dicen que los heterosexuales no corren riesgos?

Será porque estos bebes son negros,
o porque estos bebes son hispanos.

El SIDA no discrimina entre razas o nacionalidades.
¡PARE EL RACISMO! ¡LUCHE CONTRA EL SIDA!

ACT UP AIDS Coalition To Unleash Power (212) 533-8888   ACT UP is a diverse, non-partisan group of individuals united in anger and committed to direct action to end the AIDS crisis.

Gran Fury   Gran Fury is a band of individuals united in anger and committed to exploiting the power of art to end the AIDS crisis.

reassure straight people that AIDS wasn't their problem, a homophobic reassurance that also entirely denied the existence of those heterosexuals who *were* getting AIDS, primarily people of color. As Krim implied, the racism of Gould's *Cosmo* article was discernible not only in his portrayal of Africans, but also in his failure to portray what was happening to African– and Hispanic–Americans and to include them among his presumed readership. Gran Fury's poster text, in English and Spanish, therefore linked the fight against AIDS to the fight against racism.

The racist, homophobic tactic of reassuring a presumed white heterosexual audience that AIDS was not and would never become its problem belongs more consistently to the *New York Times* than any other major organ of the U.S. media. In the weeks following the demonstration against *Cosmopolitan*, the *Times* published a series of four front-page feature articles on AIDS that, typically, sought to diminish the scope of the crisis. The ACT UP collective Little Elvis responded with a simple graphic rejoinder: a crack-and-peel sticker insisting THE AIDS CRISIS IS NOT OVER. Because of the persistence of media presumptions and distortions, the sticker has unfortunately lost none of its relevance as the epidemic has been allowed to continue unabated.

AIDS: 1 in 61,
1988,
Gran Fury.
Poster, offset lithography,
22 × 17".

TRACKING THE PRESIDENTIAL COMMISSION

Metropolitan Life Insurance Building, New York City, February 15, 1988

When Ronald Reagan's Presidential Commission on the HIV Epidemic came to New York to conduct hearings in February 1988, ACT UP showed up to let commission members know angry activists were watching their every move. This was the third time ACT UP had targeted the commission. The first demonstration had been hastily organized two days after the announcement, on July 24, 1987, of those named to the commission, among whom was Cardinal John O'Connor. Because we already knew how dangerous *he* was–with his virulent homophobia and his adamant opposition to safe sex education–we chose St. Patrick's Cathedral as the site for a protest that called for O'Connor's resignation. It soon became clear that Reagan–pressured for several years by Congress and the National Academy of Sciences to establish an advisory group to help form policy on the epidemic–had sought the least informed, most biased commission he could find. Not a single one of the 14-member commission was known to have expertise about AIDS. But for the mainstream media, that wasn't a scandal. What seemed controversial to them, and to many in the administration, was the appointment of the single member who had any qualification at all: Dr. Frank Lilly, a virologist and head of genetics at Albert Einstein Medical Center, former board member of the Gay Men's Health Crisis, and . . . openly gay—hence the "controversy." Others appointed to the commission included:

- Theresa Crenshaw, a sexologist who claimed there was no such thing as safe sex, believed there was danger of contracting HIV from casual contact and supported the notorious Lyndon La Rouche ballot initiative in California requiring quarantine for those testing HIV-positive. Crenshaw's history also includes dismissal from the University of California at San Diego Medical School for misrepresenting her credentials.

- Richard M. De Vos, president of the Amway Corporation, cochairman of the Republican Leadership Council and past finance chairman of the Republican National Committee, and board member of the Robert Schuller Ministries (a televangelist corporation). With no professed knowledge of AIDS, De Vos was chosen, according to an administration spokesperson, because "we wanted to make sure we had folks on the commission with a sense for the average American."

- Cory Servaas, editor and publisher of the *Saturday Evening Post*, in which she made the claim that, working with the NIH, she had discovered a cure for AIDS. The NIH had never heard of her. She also ran a mobile AIDS testing service and was quoted as saying, "It is patriotic to have the AIDS test and be negative."

- Penny Pullen, associate of right-wing antifeminist ideologue Phyllis Schlafly and Republican leader of the Illinois State House of Representatives, where she sponsored bills requiring HIV testing for marriage license applicants and mandatory contact tracing of the sex partners of HIV-infected individuals.

- Dr. Woodrow A. Myers, Jr., Indiana State health commissioner and advocate of mandatory testing, contact tracing, and quarantine.

This "batch of geeks and unknowns," as they were characterized in the *Village Voice*, met at the National Press Building in Washington, D.C., for the first time on September 9, 1987, and ACT UP went to greet them with calls for their mass resignation. The favored chant of the day found a way to rhyme one commissioner's name with her weird solution for AIDS:

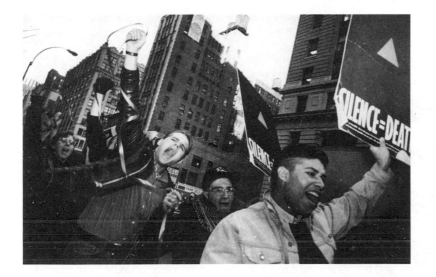

ACT UP members say "Cut the red tape" to the Presidential Commission on the HIV Epidemic at the Metropolitan Life Insurance Building, New York City, February 15, 1988 (photo: Donna Binder).

CORY SERVAAS MAKES US NERVOUS
WITH HER MOBILE TESTING SERVICE

Within three months, the commission was in total disarray. The staff director was fired, and the chairman and vice chairman resigned. The reorganized commission's new chairman, retired admiral James D. Watkins, former chief of naval operations, was again a man with no special knowledge of AIDS, but he surprised everyone–especially Ronald Reagan–with his willingness to listen to the people with genuine expertise: people working in affected communities, people with AIDS, activists. ACT UP followed the commission around the country, testifying at its hearings when possible and meeting with individual members as they grew more sympathetic. When the commission's final report was issued on June 27, 1988, its recommendations were so reasonable that President Reagan–and later President Bush–decided to ignore them.

Thus when ACT UP member Donald Moffett's HE KILLS ME poster appeared on the picket lines at the February 1988 commission hearings, it was prophetic. Targeting the smirking Reagan for his seven-year neglect of the AIDS crisis, Moffett's poster signaled to the commission and the

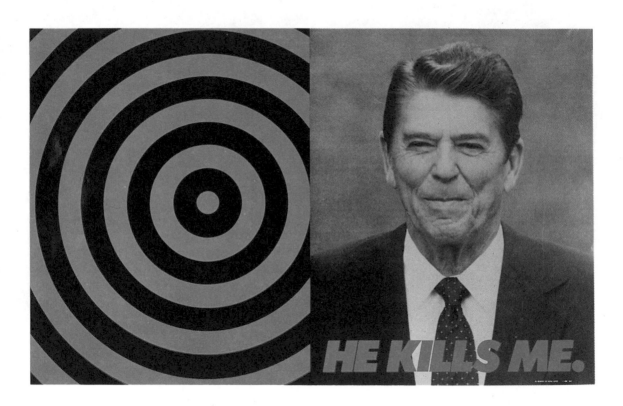

public that the president kills us in more ways than one: the laughable fool was also a murderer of people with AIDS.

Bush began his term as president by following in Reagan's footsteps, delaying the establishment of *his* AIDS commission by seven months beyond the deadline mandated by Congress. But the commission itself, this time with most members directly appointed by Congress, finally includes people who are knowledgeable about AIDS.

WALL STREET II

Wall Street, New York City, March 24, 1988

A year after ACT UP's first demonstration, we went back to Wall Street. Although we had grown enormously, learned much, and managed occasionally to make our demands known to a wide public, and although our new affinity group tactics snarled traffic in the financial district for hours and the number arrested for civil disobedience jumped from 17 to 111, the anniversary demonstration was hardly a time for celebration. New York City police were especially brutal, but we could live with that. What we couldn't live with was the persistent failure of the government to confront the crisis. Our fact sheet detailed the reasons for our frustration under the heading AFTER EIGHT YEARS OF WAITING, WE ARE **STILL** WAITING FOR:

MEDICINE

●**One year ago**, the only drug approved by the FDA for treatment against AIDS was AZT. There were eight other promising drugs, but none were available to people with AIDS.

●**One year later**, the only drug approved by the FDA for AIDS is still AZT. There are now over 40 other promising drugs, but **none** are available to people with AIDS.

FUNDING

●**One year ago**, this nation had spent less on AIDS education and research over the entire course of this epidemic than the Pentagon spent in one day.

●**One year later**, despite promises to the contrary, the federal AIDS effort is still grossly underfunded.

He Kills Me,
1987,
Donald Moffett.
Poster, offset lithography,
23⅜ × 37⅜"
(also used as placard).

Wall Street Money,
1988,
Gran Fury.
Flier, photocopy, printed
recto-verso (three versions),
3½ × 8½".

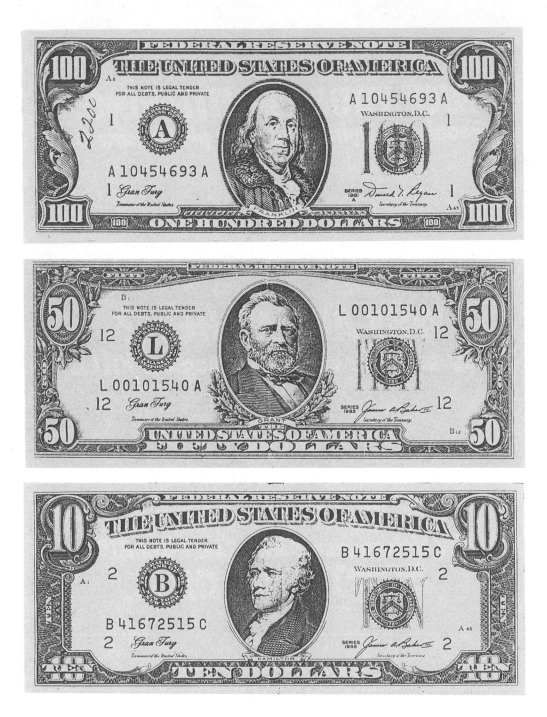

White Heterosexual Men Can't Get AIDS...
DON'T BANK ON IT.

Fight Back. Fight AIDS.

WHY ARE WE HERE?
Because your malignant neglect KILLS.

Fight Back. Fight AIDS.

FUCK YOUR PROFITEERING.
People are dying while you play business.

Fight Back. Fight AIDS.

EDUCATION

●**O n e   y e a r   a g o**, $133 million had been budgeted for AIDS education, promising a comprehensive national education program.

●**O n e   y e a r   l a t e r**, $296 million has been budgeted, and the government is still promising a national education campaign.

CIVIL RIGHTS

●**O n e   y e a r   a g o**, discrimination against people with AIDS and those suspected of having it was widespread.

●**O n e   y e a r   l a t e r**, even though civil rights protection for people with AIDS has been firmly asserted by the Supreme Court, these rights are under systematic attack by legislators, the Department of Justice, and the Civil Rights Commission.

LEADERSHIP

●**O n e   y e a r   a g o**, after 19,000 deaths, the president of the United States had not publicly acknowledged even the existence of this disease.

●**O n e   y e a r   l a t e r**, despite the fact that 80 percent of all Americans cite AIDS as the number-one health problem facing the nation today, the president still failed even to mention AIDS in his final state-of-the-union address.

AID$ Now,
1988,
Ken Woodard.
Placard, silk screen
and stencil,
18 × 24".

WALL STREET II inspired a number of new graphic interventions. Gran Fury photocopied thousands of $10, $50, and $100 bills to be scattered in the streets, each with caustic words directed at Wall Street brokers on its back. And the simple AID$ NOW placard, generic enough to be used in many demonstrations to come, appeared along with SILENCE = DEATH and AIDS-GATE among the ranks blocking downtown business-as-usual traffic.

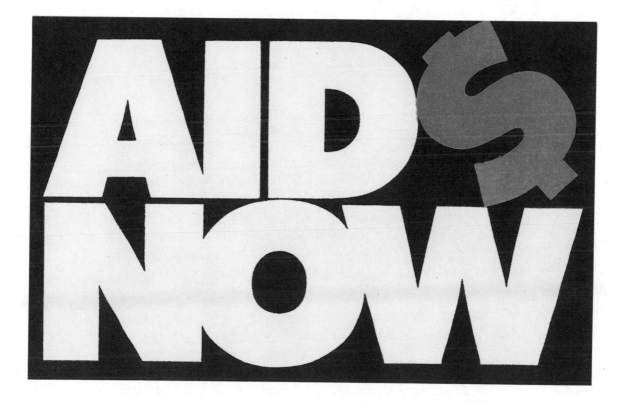

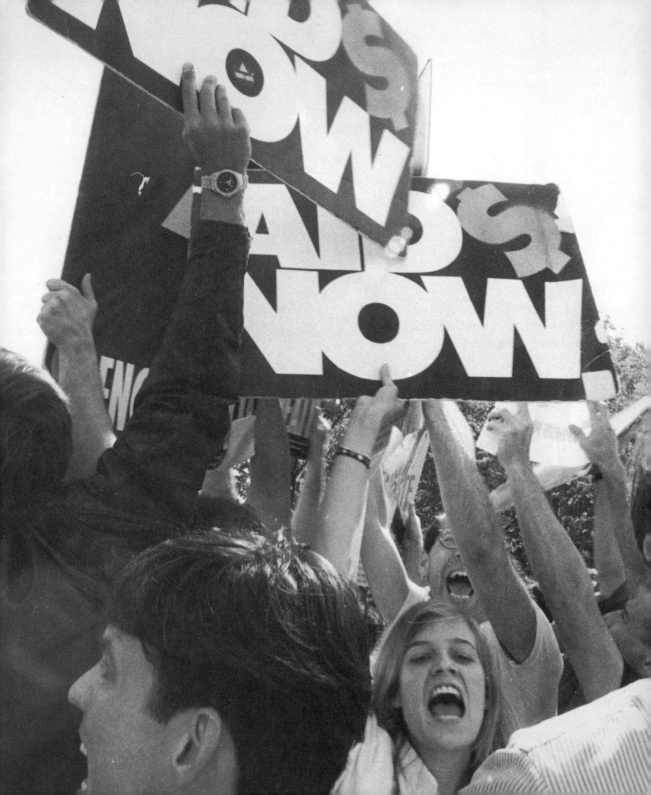

NINE DAYS OF PROTEST

Various locations in New York City; Newark, New Jersey; and Albany, New York, April 29–May 7, 1988

The first nationally coordinated action of the AIDS Coalition to Network, Organize, and Win (ACT NOW)—a national association of AIDS activist groups formed during the 1987 March on Washington for Lesbian and Gay Rights—took place around the United States on nine days in the spring of 1988. ACT NOW suggested, but did not dictate, issues to be addressed separately on each of the days, and individual AIDS activist groups determined both the local issues of greatest importance and the nature of the demonstrations to confront them. ACT UP New York focused, on consecutive days, on homophobia, people with AIDS, people of color, substance abuse, prisons, women, the worldwide crisis, and testing and treatment, and we went to Albany for ACT NOW's national day of protest at state legislatures.

Gran Fury produced a series of photocopied posters, wheatpasted around New York, to announce ACT UP's demonstrations. These included an overall call to action stating ALL PEOPLE WITH AIDS ARE INNOCENT, meant to combat the mainstream media's division of people with AIDS into "innocent victims"—infants, hemophiliacs, and transfusion-related cases—and, by implication, guilty victims—gay people, IV drug users, sex workers, and so on. The statement appears in conjunction with a caduceus, the medical profession's chosen symbol, and thus demands of health care professionals that they live up to their purported ethical standard of equal and compassionate treatment for all, including all people with AIDS.

Among Gran Fury's most popular and durable images are the two posters produced for the same-sex kiss-in, in protest of homophobic responses to AIDS. One used a World War II photograph of kissing sailors, the other a lesbian couple from a 1920s Broadway play, and both carried the embedded text READ MY LIPS (Gran Fury beat George Bush to the punch in using the line). ACT UP women objected to the sexual difference marked by the two images—men aggressively kissing, women staring longingly into each other's eyes—because it reinforced the stereotype of desexualized lesbian desire compared with sexy gay male desire. When Gran Fury made T-shirts of the kiss-in images, they righted the imbalance by using a historical image of lesbians kissing.

Photo: Ben Thornberry

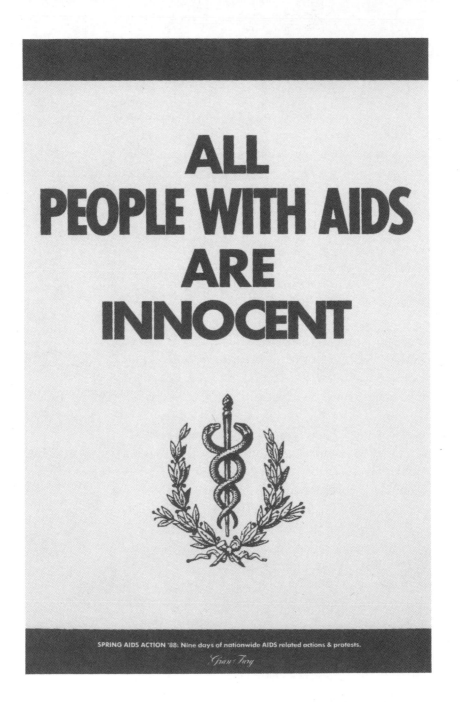

ALL
PEOPLE WITH AIDS
ARE
INNOCENT

SPRING AIDS ACTION '88: Nine days of nationwide AIDS related actions & protests.

Gran Fury

The controversy over the degree of sexualization in the Gran Fury images was directly relevant to the event–a public demonstration and celebration of gay and lesbian sexuality in the face of homophobia. As the fact sheet headed WHY WE KISS stated:

● **We kiss** in an aggressive demonstration of affection.

● **We kiss** to protest the cruel and painful bigotry that affects the lives of lesbians and gay men.

● **We kiss** so that all who see us will be forced to confront their own homophobia.

● **We kiss** to challenge repressive conventions that prohibit displays of love between persons of the same sex.

● **We kiss** as an affirmation of our feelings, our desires, ourselves.

The flier went on to detail facts about homophobia and its linkage to AIDS:

● One in ten lesbians and one in five gay men have been physically assaulted because of their sexuality.

● The Helms Amendment, preventing federal funding of any AIDS educational materials that could be construed to promote lesbian or gay sex, passed in the Senate by a vote of 96 to 2.

● The federal government has been unconscionably slow to react to the AIDS crisis, a slowness tantamount to condoning the deaths of tens of thousands of gay men.

● The Civil Rights Commission is opposing legislation authorizing the gathering of bias-related crime statistics because it objects to the inclusion of sexual orientation as a bias category. This is despite its own admission that crimes against gay men and women, aggravated by perceptions about AIDS, are probably the most widespread hate-crimes today.

On April 30, day two of the nationally coordinated actions, ACT UP New York combined forces with ACT UP New Jersey to confront University Hospital in Newark over its neglect of the needs of people with AIDS. Essex County, New Jersey, where Newark is located, had reported 1,154 cases of AIDS, the vast majority of them drug-related. One in 20 babies was

All People with AIDS Are Innocent,
1988,
Gran Fury.
Poster, offset lithography,
16¼ × 10½".

Read My Lips (boys),
1988,
Gran Fury.
Poster, offset lithography,
16¼ × 10¾"
(also used as T-shirt).

Read My Lips (girls),
1988,
Gran Fury.
Poster, offset lithography,
16½ × 10⅛"
(variant used as T-shirt).

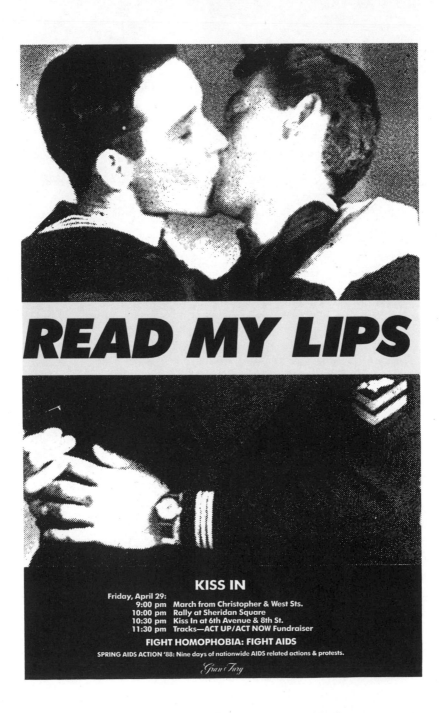

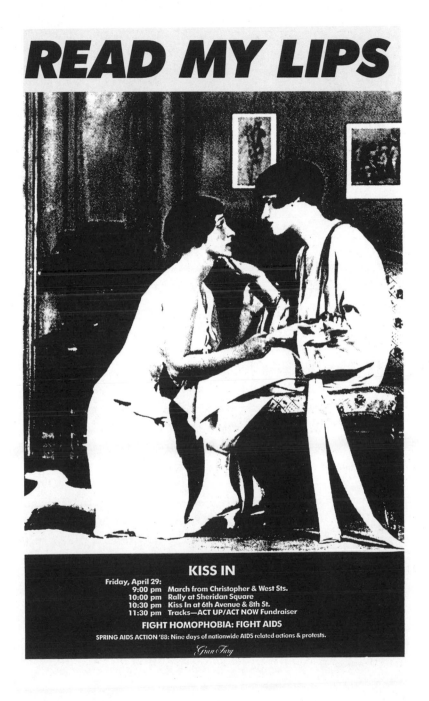

being born HIV-positive. Because this was an impoverished population, its only access to experimental drugs was through clinical trials, and yet the main hospital treating these people was not conducting any. ACT UP demanded that:

- University Hospital, Newark, commence offering clinical trials using the most promising experimental drugs, not just AZT, which is too toxic for many people with AIDS.

- University Hospital provide its HIV-infected patients with a list of clinical trials available in nearby New York.

- New Jersey allocate research funds to expand enrollment in clinical trials and to increase the number of drugs offered.

AIDS in communities of color had become a sensitive issue for ACT UP. We were, after all, a mostly white, mostly middle-class, mostly gay group. Originally an Outreach Committee attempted to build bridges to organizations—the Minority Task Force on AIDS, the Hispanic AIDS Forum, the Association for Drug Abuse Prevention and Treatment—working in other affected communities, mostly nonwhite, mostly poor, mostly—but certainly not always—straight. Eventually we formed our own Majority Actions Committee, so named because the majority of people with AIDS in New York are people of color and because the word *minority* is rejected by those very people as reinforcing their marginal status.

On the third day of the spring actions, with the endorsement of Reverend Jesse Jackson, ACT UP members reached out to New York's Black and Hispanic churches to solicit their commitment to fighting AIDS. A flier drawn up for the action quoted from an important document prepared by the AIDS Discrimination Unit of the New York City Commission on Human Rights called AIDS AND PEOPLE OF COLOR: THE DISCRIMINATORY IMPACT:

- People of color, already burdened by a history of racism and economic disparity, have borne a tremendous share of the AIDS crisis.

- In New York City, 55 percent of all persons with AIDS are Black or Hispanic. This figure is greater than the 44 percent population figure for Blacks and Hispanics living in New York City.

- On the national level, the statistical gap is even wider. While Blacks comprise only 12 percent of the total population, more than 24 percent of those with AIDS in the United States are Black. Similarly Hispanics, who comprise only 6 percent of our national population, represent 14 percent of all people with AIDS in the United States.

A letter to church pastors offered the assistance of ACT UP members in planning and carrying out AIDS awareness programs and asked them to consider:

- Addressing the issue in a sermon or during a period of prayer and meditation.

- Planning a special presentation during or after worship by the church's social-action committee.

- Collecting a special offering to further the work of AIDS service and advocacy groups in communities of color.

- Setting up a special booth or table during pre- or postworship fellowship hour at which members of the congregation might receive information about AIDS and sign petitions calling on Black and Hispanic caucuses of the New York State Legislature and the U.S. Congress to hold hearings on the issue of AIDS and its impact on people of color.

For the day devoted to AIDS and substance abuse, ACT UP teamed up with the Association for Drug Abuse Prevention and Treatment (ADAPT) for a noontime rally at City Hall. Demands were spelled out by ADAPT, the primary nongovernmental organization working with IV drug users in the city and a vocal proponent of a needle-exchange program like the one that had been so successful in reducing HIV transmission among intravenous drug users in Amsterdam. In addition to a demand for free needles, ACT UP and ADAPT called for the expansion of drug treatment and street outreach prevention programs and the development of housing for people with AIDS. These demands were made in light of daunting statistics listed on the fact sheet:

- There are 250,000 intravenous drug users (IVDUs) in New York City. Three years ago 10 percent of the city's IVDUs had been exposed to HIV. Now in 1988 over 60 percent have been exposed.

- There are 1,400 women with AIDS in New York City. Eighty percent were IVDUs or had sex with an IVDU. Eighty-four percent are Black or Hispanic.

- One thousand HIV-antibody-positive babies are expected to be born this year in New York City. Ninety-four percent of children with AIDS are Black or Hispanic. In 82 percent of pediatric cases of AIDS, one or both parents were IVDUs.

- Drug users are reported to account for 70 percent of AIDS patients in New York City municipal hospitals, and almost all cases of AIDS in prison involve inmates with histories of IV drug use.

At the same time: THE LAST DRUG TREATMENT PROGRAM TO OPEN IN NEW YORK CITY WAS IN 1972. One of Mayor Ed Koch's "solutions" to the so-called fiscal crisis of the mid-1970s was to transfer all responsibility for drug treatment to the state. The result was effectively the abandonment of all efforts to help people get off drugs. That, in conjunction with no real commitment to needle exchange or clean "works" education, has meant that the city has virtually ensured the HIV infection of its large—and growing—IV drug-using population.

On May 3, ACT UP gathered at the Harlem State Office Building, which houses the State Office of Corrections, to protest the treatment of people with AIDS (PWAs) in prisons. We condemned as CRUEL AND UNUSUAL PUNISHMENT the state's practice of segregating and even shackling incarcerated PWAs, thus stigmatizing them among their fellow prisoners and allowing them no access to recreation, education, and work release. Prisoners diagnosed with AIDS die twice as fast as PWAs outside of prison, owing to poor health care or, in some cases, none at all. And in spite of the known incidence of drug use and sex among prisoners, the state refused to provide either education or condoms, thus increasing the already alarming rate of HIV infection among the prison population. ACT UP therefore demanded:

- Adequate health care in prison—decent facilities, access to all therapeutic treatments, a full staff of competent and compassionate health care workers.

- No segregation of or discrimination against people with AIDS or ARC or persons testing positive or perceived to be at risk for AIDS. End the shackling of prisoners with AIDS.

AIDS Behind Bars,
1988,
Gran Fury.
Poster, offset lithography,
16⅞ × 10⅞".

25% TEST POSITIVE

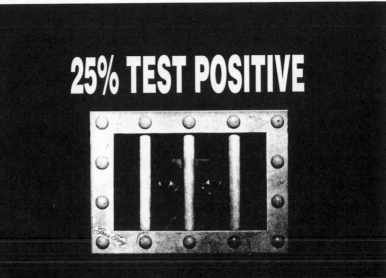

People with AIDS in prison live 1/2
as long as those treated outside.
Let's put AIDS education and treatment behind bars.

Prison authorities know that effective
AIDS education, condoms and dental
dams reduce risk, yet these are not
available to prisoners in N.Y. State.
To protest this callous negligence,
send a condom to Marion Borum,
Deputy Director for Program Services,
N.Y.S. Dept. of Corrections, State Office Campus, Building 2, Albany, N.Y.
12226

Join us in protest on Tuesday May 3rd
at 4 PM at the offices for the New York
State Department of Correction, Harlem State Building, 125th St. at Adam
Clayton Powell Blvd. Speakers will
include Yolanda Serrano of ADAPT and
Billy Jones of the Whitman Walker Clinic.

● Comprehensive, effective, and ongoing education for prisoners and correction officers.

● Explicit safe sex and safe "works" education and distribution of clean "works," condoms, and dental dams in prisons.

● No forced testing of prisoners for HIV infection. Counseling and support for prisoners with AIDS and their families. Medical and compassionate parole and release programs. Appointment of an ombudsperson at the state level to coordinate an effective, humane policy regarding HIV infection among prisoners.

On May 4, ACT UP staged two actions directed at women's issues, both organized by ACT UP's Women's Committee and both focusing on sexual transmission. During the day, ACT UP members took sexually explicit AIDS prevention materials, condoms, dental dams, lubricants, and jellies to New York City high schools to provide lifesaving information to teenagers. Working in teams of two or three outside of nine different schools, ACT UP members talked to eager students about safe sex, showed them how to use the condoms and dams, and gave away everything they'd brought in short order. Apart from the direct intervention, the action also implicitly functioned as a protest of the board of education's refusal to give young people explicit safe sex information, even though the education authorities know that large numbers of young people are very much at risk for and are becoming infected with HIV. The city's failure to educate teenagers about AIDS was due in large measure to the unholy alliance between the city's oddest and most reactionary couple–Mayor Koch and Cardinal O'Connor–to whose duel "leadership" can certainly be attributed thousands of New York City AIDS deaths.

In the evening, ACT UP went to Shea Stadium in Queens for a Mets game. In a gutsy attempt to get straight men to take responsibility for the health of their sex partners–official advice about safe sex practices is almost always directed at *women*–activists handed out information and condoms and unfurled banners in the three blocks of seats we occupied–400 seats in three different sections of the stadium. The banners bore such slogans as STRIKE OUT AIDS, NO GLOVE NO LOVE, and DON'T BALK AT SAFER SEX. A flier distributed to the baseball fans under the rubric AIDS IS NO BALL GAME contained a scorecard:

Sexism Rears Its
Unprotected Head,
1988,
Gran Fury.
Poster, offset lithography,
16⅛ × 10⅛".

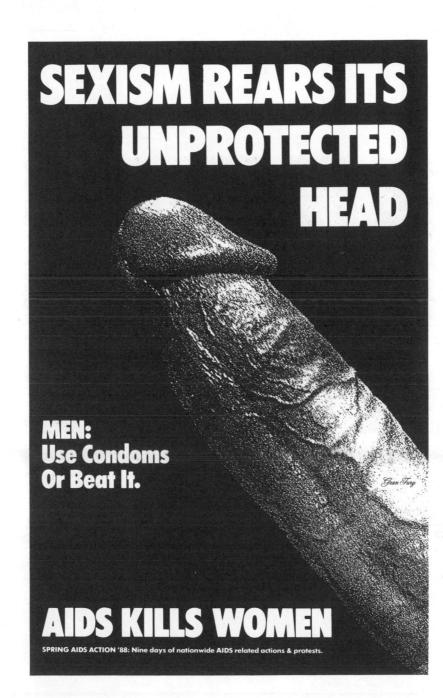

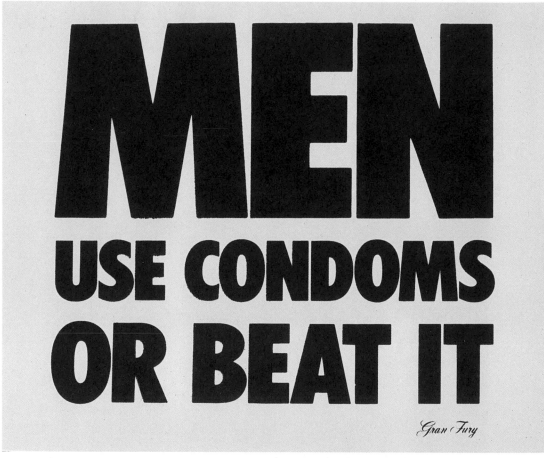

SINGLE Only **o n e** woman has been included in government-sponsored tests for new drugs for AIDS.

DOUBLE Women diagnosed with AIDS die **t w i c e** as fast as men.

TRIPLE The number of women with AIDS has **t r i p l e d** as a result of sexual contact with men in New York City since the 1984 World Series.

THE
GRAND Most men **s t i l l** don't use condoms.
SLAM

In conjunction with the AIDS and Women day, but for obvious reasons not used at the demonstration sites, Gran Fury produced their most **g r a p h i c** design, as well as one of their most memorable phrases: MEN, USE CONDOMS OR BEAT IT. This phrase was catchy enough to demand reissue, so the collective printed a crack-and-peel sticker with the phrase in boldface type on a fluorescent background; later the design was printed on a T-shirt and, under the auspices of the Gay Men's Health Crisis, as a button.

On May 5, ACT UP held a rally at the International Building at Rockefeller Center to call attention to AIDS as a worldwide crisis. A fact sheet demanded that the U.S. government provide world leadership, pay its $113 million back dues to the World Health Organization (WHO), increase its contribution to WHO's special AIDS program, increase aid to Africa, cease mandatory HIV testing, and develop a comprehensive AIDS policy. As the nation most affected by AIDS, the United States has not only failed to assume leadership in combatting the epidemic, but also acted in open defiance of most of the World Health Organization's recommendations. The fact sheet contrasted the two positions:

WHO RECOMMENDATIONS

- Education, not mandatory testing, is the best defense against AIDS.

- All people in the world must be informed of the need to use condoms and how to avoid the risks of IV drug use.

- There is no public health rationale to justify isolation, quarantine, or other discriminatory measures based solely on a person's HIV infection status or practice of risk behaviors.

Men, Use Condoms
or Beat It,
1988,
Gran Fury.
Crack-and-peel sticker,
silk screen,
7⅛ × 8⅝"
(also used as T-shirt
and button).

U.S. RESPONSE

● The United States uses tests for HIV infection to exclude immigrants, isolate prisoners, and discriminate against military and state department personnel.

● Three years after Congress appropriated funds to educate all Americans about AIDS, the federal government still has no comprehensive national education program.

WHO RECOMMENDATIONS

● We must provide humane care to people with AIDS and provide counseling and social support and services to people infected with HIV.

● We must have the strength to reject simplistic solutions for AIDS control, and the will to ensure participation of the entire health and social sector in an active program **against AIDS – for health**.

U.S. RESPONSE

● The United States and South Africa are the only two industrialized countries where you can be denied health care because of lack of money.

Liberty and Justice for All[*],
1988
(produced for U.S. Civil
Rights Commission
demonstration, 1988),
Ken Woodard.
Flier, photocopy,
11 × 8½"

● People who are HIV-infected can be denied health insurance.

● Reagan's Civil Rights Commission is threatening to take away the civil rights of people infected with HIV.

WHO RECOMMENDATIONS

● We must open fully the channels of international communications and encourage the exchange of scientific information on AIDS research.

U.S. RESPONSE

● The Food and Drug Administration refuses to accept research from other countries on promising new drug therapies. Americans have to travel to other countries for treatment.

The following day, devoted to testing and treatment issues, ACT UP moved up Fifth Avenue to the world's most famous toy store. F.A.O. Schwarz was chosen as a symbol of the lavish amount of money spent on the children of the rich, while not so far away hundreds of impoverished infants with AIDS languish in public hospitals with inadequate care. The specific target of the demonstration, detailed on a fact sheet, was the first federally funded clinical trial for pediatric AIDS, then under way in 30

LIBERTY AND JUSTICE FOR ALL*

*Offer not available to anyone with AIDS

NINE DAYS OF PROTEST

hospitals around the country. The trial was for the efficacy of intravenous immunoglobulin (IVIG). In spite of the fact that the drug was already approved for certain pediatric immunodeficiencies and was being used by many doctors treating infants with AIDS, the government devised a testing protocol requiring that half the babies receive placebos. Using placebos instead of drugs for terminal illnesses is unethical in any case, but using a placebo in an invasive procedure is doubly life-threatening. Administered intravenously every 28 days for up to eight hours, the drug—or the placebo—often requires restraining the child (the median age of the trial participants was 18 months). Worse still, there is high risk of infection from the procedure itself, which could thus actually *cause* the baby's death. But because the vast majority of pediatric AIDS cases are among poor Blacks and Hispanics, their only possibility of receiving the drug is by entering a drug trial. ACT UP's flier concluded:

- The protocol for this drug trial should be rewritten to remove the placebo.

- No AIDS drug trials, or any trial of drugs that may offer hope to patients suffering from life-threatening diseases for which there is no alternative treatment, should employ placebos.

- All human beings whose lives are threatened by injury or illness should have equal access to the drugs and treatments that can save their lives. Good health care is a basic human right.

The ninth day of protest saw ACT UP in Albany for a display of New York panels of the Names Project quilt in Washington Park, followed by a march and rally at the state capital, where ACT UP member and PWA Vito Russo addressed the gathered crowd about New York State's inaction on AIDS. Though the largest concentration of HIV infection is in New York City, many of the programs to fight AIDS must be state-funded, and thus Governor Mario Cuomo and the state legislature are culpable for many of the city's inadequacies. In a flier titled WE DEMAND A STATE OF EMERGENCY, ACT UP insisted on the following measures:

- Immediate passage of the New York State Bias Crime legislation empowering the prosecution of hate violence against lesbians and gay men.

68 | 69

- The creation of affordable housing, adequate support services, and skilled nursing facilities for people with AIDS, and quality care for PWAs in hospitals throughout New York State.

- Culturally sensitive, sex positive, and nonhomophobic AIDS education, which must also reflect heterosexual male responsibility.

- Massive increases in funding for drug rehabilitation, and availability of culturally appropriate syringe sterilization education.

- Appointment by the New York State Department of Corrections of an independent advocate for the rights of prisoners to comprehensive health care services; distribution of condoms and dental dams in prisons; full access of prisoners to drug rehabilitation programs.

Photo: T. L. Litt

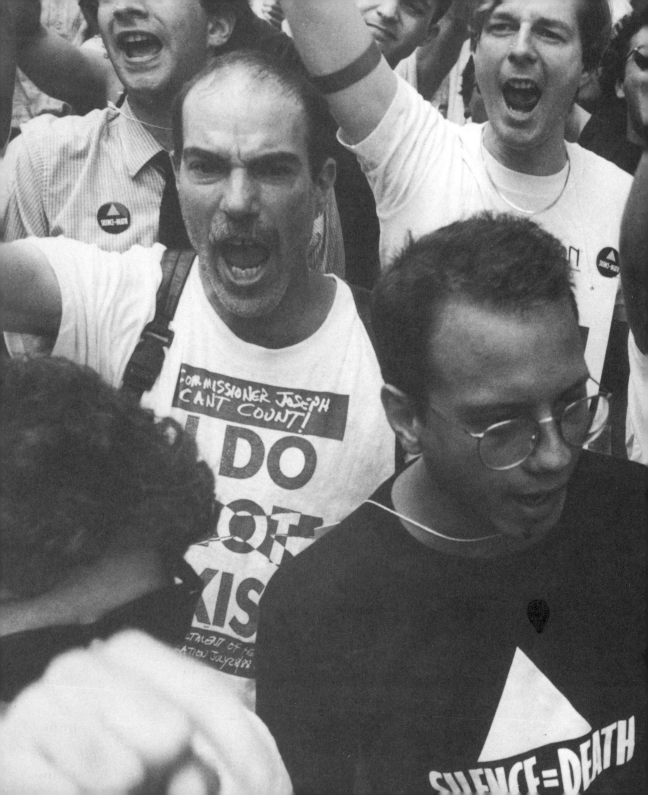

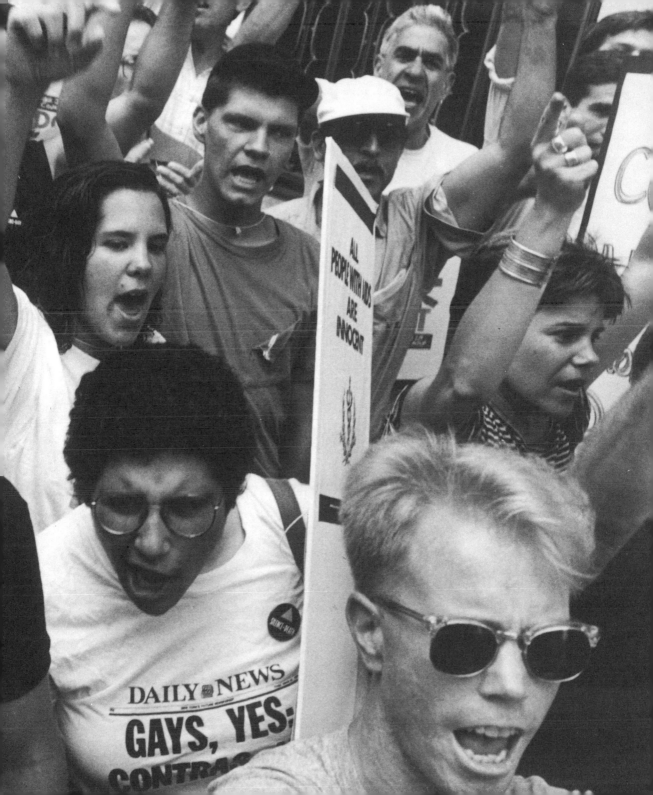

New York City Department of Health, July 28, 1988

New York City health commissioner Stephen Joseph became the enemy of the communities affected by AIDS from the moment of his appointment on May 5, 1986. True, his was a tough job—defending his boss Mayor Koch's unwillingness to spend city money to combat the epidemic, but he did more than that. ACT UP's first serious run-in with Joseph was over one of his first public positions on AIDS: considering out loud "mandatory AIDS testing for prostitutes and sex and drug offenders, as well as a heavy crackdown on all forms of prostitution." It was a standard failed public health policy: look and act tough, scapegoat and punish the most feared and disenfranchised populations. On December 10, 1987, an ACT UP affinity group calling itself the Metropolitan Health Association (MHA) made an appointment to see Joseph. Once in his office, they refused to leave until Joseph agreed to reconsider his position. Eight MHA members were arrested and charged with trespass. Joseph's love of "AIDS testing" and his contempt for AIDS activists and everyone else working in the affected communities would only intensify in his two remaining years in office.

In the summer of 1988, Joseph showed just how cynical he could be when it came to justifying the city's lack of commitment to meeting the needs of people with AIDS. Long-range funding requirements for AIDS in New York City had been based on a 1986 calculation of 400,000 people infected with HIV. At that time, it was thought that only 50 percent of infected individuals would ultimately develop AIDS. Two years later, however, it was understood that, untreated, virtually everyone infected would eventually become ill. And this meant that the city's funding projections were drastically inadequate. For example, Deputy State Comptroller Elinor Bachrach criticized the city's estimated need for 2,703 hospital beds for AIDS patients in 1991, stating that in fact the city would require an average of 6,400 beds. On July 19, Joseph responded with a quick statistical fix: he simply cut the New York City estimates in half, claiming now that only 200,000 were infected. His new arithmetic was informed by no epidemiology at all (the city had done no primary epidemiological research), but rather by comparing apples to oranges. Joseph's cut was mostly achieved by reducing the number of New York City's gay men presumed infected from 200,000 to 50,000, based on a comparison with infection rates among gay men in San Francisco and an absurdly low estimate of New York's gay male population at 100,000. Joseph ignored a number of facts regarding men who have sex with men in the two cities. San Francisco's gay community is far more homogeneous and better organized and informed about AIDS than is New York's. Because of class, racial, and ethnic differences between the two cities' populations of men who have sex with men, the percentage of these men who identify themselves as members of a gay community and thus have access to community-based AIDS education is drastically different. Thus the decline in new HIV infections among gay men in San Francisco is far greater than it is in New York, where Joseph's health department had made no effort to get safe sex information to men engaged in risky same-sex sexual activity.

On July 28, ACT UP staged a demonstration and sit-in at the New York City Department of Health (DOH) to protest Joseph's faked epidemiology. And Gran Fury came up with a citywide guerrilla graphic blitz. They printed a poster with a bloody hand print and the caption YOU'VE GOT BLOOD ON YOUR HANDS, STEPHEN JOSEPH. THE CUT IN AIDS NUMBERS IS A LETHAL LIE. An alternative bloody-hand poster read YOU'VE GOT BLOOD ON YOUR HANDS, ED KOCH. NYC AIDS CARE DOESN'T EXIST. These were wheat-pasted on hoardings, mail boxes, telephone booths—wherever a flat surface existed. Simultaneously, crews of ACT UP members went about with buckets of red paint, into which they dipped their latex-glove-covered hands to imprint bloody palm prints all over the city.

When 11 members of an ACT UP affinity group were arrested for disrupting a meeting at the health commissioner's office the following week, ACT UP decided to hound Joseph wherever he went. A series of phone zaps of the health department and interruptions of his public appearances came to be known in the group as SURRENDER DOROTHY: our obsession with getting this man out of office had turned us into a collective Wicked Witch of the West. But we soon learned who was really Dorothy and who the witch, when Joseph's vindictiveness toward people who opposed his policies resulted in aggressive prosecution and conviction of the 11 ACT UP members who had occupied the DOH office.

Nearly a year after Joseph's statistical wishing away of gay New Yorkers, he once again defied the collective wisdom of public health officials and community-based organizations working against the spread of AIDS. During a plenary session of the Fifth International Conference on

AIDS in Montreal in June 1989, Joseph called for mandatory name reporting and contact tracing of the sex partners of people testing HIV-positive. He claimed that this was now necessitated by the fact that immune-system monitoring and early treatment intervention for those who are HIV-positive could prolong and perhaps save their lives. Members of ACT UP attending the conference immediately called Joseph to account at an impromptu press conference after his speech, and the next day, June 8, 200 ACT UP members disrupted early morning traffic on the Brooklyn Bridge and temporarily shut down the nearby health department building. Shouting FIRST YOU DON'T EXIST, NOW YOU'RE ON HIS LIST, ACT UP members distributed fliers announcing STEPHEN JOSEPH WANTS YOUR NAME:

WHAT'S WRONG WITH THIS PICTURE
- Joseph says that if names are kept, better follow-up and treatment could be administered. If nine years into the AIDS crisis New York City cannot provide the most basic services, how does Joseph think the city can provide the "luxury" of adequate treatment?

- Those who are most at risk will be driven underground, afraid of being stigmatized, thrown out of their homes and jobs, with no available treatment options.

TRACING IS NOT A CURE FOR AIDS
- The Centers for Disease Control estimate that the cost of tracing per person is $5,000 to $7,000. With Joseph estimating 200,000 people to be HIV-infected, the cost of contact tracing for New York City alone could be 1.4 billion dollars.

NO LISTING, NO TRACING, NO WAY!
We demand:
- That Mayor Koch denounce Joseph's plan for routine contact tracing and confidential rather than anonymous testing.

- That Mayor Koch fire Stephen Joseph and hire a competent health commissioner, knowledgeable of HIV-related illnesses and services and with proven experience in dealing with the communities affected by AIDS.

- That anonymous HIV testing and counseling sites be maintained and expanded, to serve all affected communities in all boroughs.

- That treatments be made available to everyone with HIV-related illnesses and

Deadlier than the Virus,
1989,
Richard Deagle.
Subway advertising poster,
offset lithography,
10¾ × 16⅜".

DEADLIER THAN THE VIRUS

STEPHEN C. JOSEPH
COMMISSIONER OF HEALTH, NYC

that aggressive education and counseling on treatment options, safe sex, and safe needle use be instituted.

When it became clear that virtually every AIDS service and advocacy organization in the city agreed with ACT UP in opposing Joseph's proposal, Koch—now fearing for his political career—was forced to block it.

In the late fall of 1989, during the transition from Koch's mayoralty to that of David Dinkins, Stephen Joseph resigned his position as health commissioner. But not without a parting insult to those of us in the affected communities with whom he had always failed to consult: once again, and now with a pretense of the full support of the New York City Board of Health, Joseph asked the state health department to collect the names of people who test positive for HIV and to trace and contact their sex partners and those with whom they shared needles.

SEIZE CONTROL OF THE FDA

Food and Drug Administration Headquarters, Rockville, Maryland, October 11, 1988

Time Isn't the Only Thing the FDA Is Killing,
1988,
Ken Woodard.
Placard, offset lithography,
24 × 18".

Our takeover of the FDA was unquestionably the most significant demonstration of the AIDS activist movement's first two years. Organized nationally by ACT NOW to take place on the anniversary of the March on Washington for Lesbian and Gay Rights and just following the second Washington showing of the Names Project quilt, the protest began with a Columbus Day rally at the Department of Health and Human Services under the banner HEALTH CARE IS A RIGHT and proceeded the following morning to a siege of FDA headquarters in a Washington suburb.

If "drugs into bodies" had been central to ACT UP from the beginning, the protest at the FDA represented both a culmination of our early efforts and a turning point in both recognition by the government of the seriousness and legitimacy of our demands and national awareness of the AIDS activist movement. This turning point occurred for two interrelated reasons: 1) the demonstrated knowledge by AIDS activists of every detail of the complex FDA drug approval process, and 2) a professionally designed campaign that prepared the media to convey our treatment issues to the public.

The entire body of ACT UP was schooled in advance with knowledge of

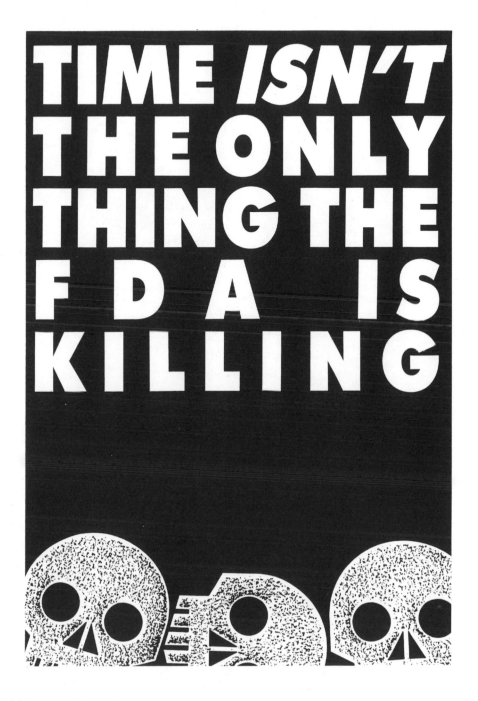

complicated issues that until then had largely remained the province of Treatment and Data Committee members. The latter, who had been studying treatment issues for over a year and had also profited from knowledge garnered by AIDS activists in other U.S. cities, prepared an FDA ACTION HANDBOOK of more than 40 pages and conducted a series of teach-ins for ACT UP's general membership. This information was then distilled by the Media Committee for presentation to the press. The FDA action was "sold" in advance to the media almost like a Hollywood movie, with a carefully prepared and presented press kit, hundreds of phone calls to members of the press, and activists' appearances scheduled on television and radio talk shows around the country. When the demonstration took place, the media were not only there to get the story, they knew what that story was, and they reported it with a degree of accuracy and sympathy that is, to say the least, unusual.

ACT UP's fundamental contention was that, with a new epidemic disease such as AIDS, testing experimental new therapies is itself a form of health care and that access to health care must be everyone's right. Although Reagan conservatives and pharmaceutical companies attempted to co-opt our agenda, our demands were very different from their profit-driven desire for deregulation. AIDS activists want *consumer* interests protected, not the profits of pharmaceutical companies. We want drugs proven safe and effective, but we want them faster, and we want them equally access-

Members of ACT UP's Majority Actions Committee at FDA headquarters, Rockville, Maryland, October 11, 1988 (photo: Donna Binder).

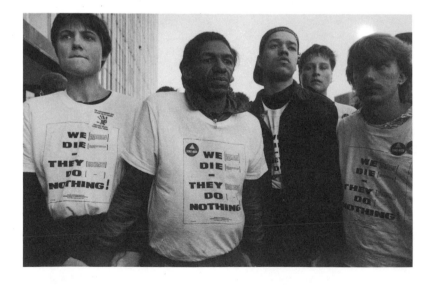

ible for everyone who needs them. Our demands to the FDA included the following:

- Shorten the drug approval process. The FDA must ensure immediate free access to drugs proven safe and theoretically effective—that is, as soon as Phase I trials are completed—together with clear information that the drug has not yet been proven effective.

- No more double-blind placebo trials. Because giving a placebo to someone with a life-threatening illness is unethical, the FDA must inform designers of clinical trials that it will not accept data based on placebo trials. Instead, new drugs must be measured against other approved drugs or, where there are none, against other experimental therapies, different doses of the same drug, or against what is already known of the natural progression of AIDS.

- Allowance of concurrent prophylaxis. The FDA must accept no new drug trials that prohibit simultaneously taking another drug to prevent opportunistic infections; it must also allow concurrent prophylaxis in any ongoing trials and insist that researchers inform trial participants of their right to use preventive, lifesaving treatments.

- Include people from all affected populations at all stages of HIV infection in clinical trials. The FDA must mandate that drug trials recruit participants from all groups affected by HIV infection, including women, people of color, children, poor people, IV drug users, hemophiliacs, and gay men. If a trial requires a homogeneous population, parallel trials must be conducted in other affected populations. Moreover, trials must be opened to people at all stages of HIV infection, not simply those with CDC-defined AIDS.

- The FDA must set clear criteria for proving the safety and efficacy of a drug and coordinate drug trials in order to prevent drug companies from wasting time with new or redundant trials.

- Institutional Review Boards designed to protect trial participants must be broadened to include people with HIV infection or their informed advocates.

- The FDA must release all potentially lifesaving information—for example, follow-up data on already-approved drugs now in use—no matter what information drug companies believe they own. The FDA must also keep a computerized registry of all clinical trials and make it available to people with HIV

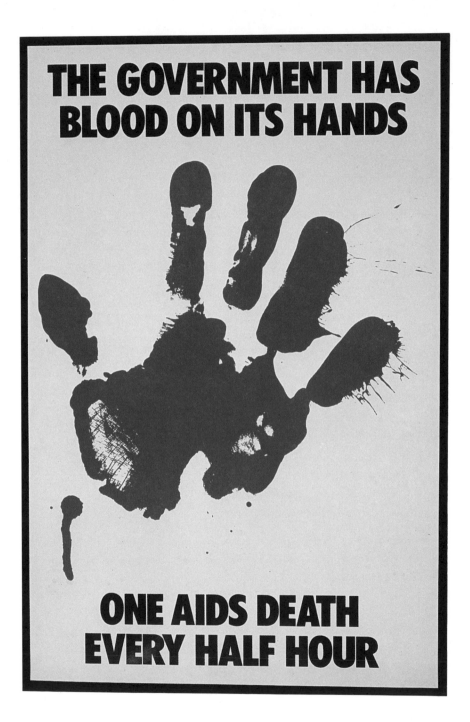

infection and their doctors. Preliminary results of trials must be made available to participants throughout the trial so that they can make their own health care decisions.

- The FDA must rewrite the criteria for investigational new drugs (INDs) to include anyone who is HIV-infected, and drug companies must be compelled to release drugs through the IND program. Until the FDA has been given the power to do that, it must release any information concerning new drugs so that AIDS activists can pressure drug companies to apply for an IND designation.

- Medicaid and private health insurance must be made to pay for experimental drug therapies.

- The FDA must support rather than harass community groups working to keep community members alive by conducting community-based research and operating buyers' clubs—in other words, trying to do what the federal bureaucracy has thus far failed to do.

These demands, whose articulateness stemmed from in-depth knowledge of the history and workings of the drug approval bureaucracy, formed the background to ACT NOW's civil disobedience at FDA headquarters. Affinity groups from around the country engaged all day in skirmishes with the Rockville police, who had clearly been ordered to keep the number of arrests low to minimize media drama. When we blocked the departure of buses full of arrestees (176 activists did manage to provoke arrest), they dragged us out of the street and left us sitting in the grass. When we tried to enter the building, they forcibly restrained us, but refused to arrest us. We did, though, manage to stop business as usual, to occupy FDA headquarters at least symbolically. ACT UP graphics and banners covered the building's facade, and demonstrators staged one piece of theater after another as the television cameras rolled on.

Most affinity groups improvised their own costumes and props for the occasion. ACT UP's Majority Actions Committee made a reproducible design for T-shirts and posters, WE DIE—THEY DO NOTHING, spelling out in fine print who WE are [People of color, whether we are Afro-American, Native American, Hispanic Latino, or Asian, women, men, IV drug users, partners of IV drug users, lesbians, gays, straights, the homeless, prisoners, and children affected by the AIDS crisis], who THEY are [Ronald Reagan, George Bush, Michael Dukakis, the NIH, the FDA, the U.S. Congress, the

The Government Has Blood on Its Hands,
1988,
Gran Fury.
Poster, offset lithography,
31¾ × 21⅛"
(also used as placard,
crack-and-peel sticker,
and T-shirt).

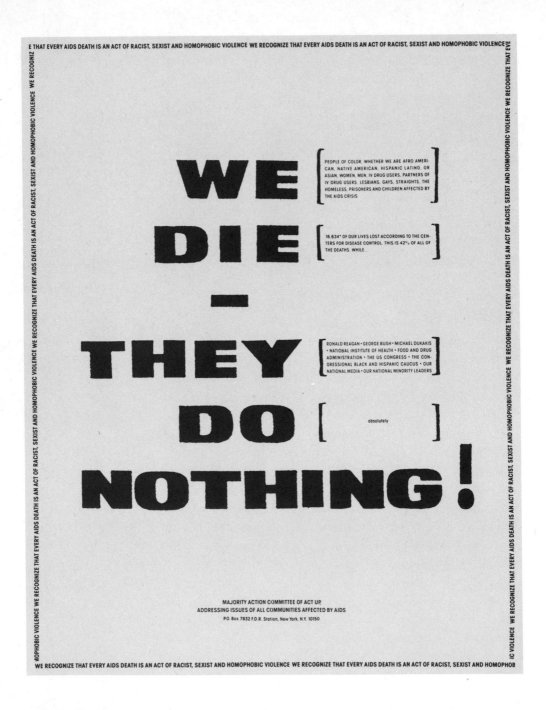

Congressional Black and Hispanic Caucus, our national media, our national minority leaders], and declaring, around the border, WE RECOGNIZE EVERY AIDS DEATH AS AN ACT OF RACIST, SEXIST, AND HOMOPHOBIC VIOLENCE. Gran Fury reworked an earlier image–the bloody hand–for placards, stickers, and T-shirts. The bloodied hand print that had initially appeared to protest New York City health commissioner Stephen Joseph's cut in projected AIDS cases now said THE GOVERNMENT HAS BLOOD ON ITS HANDS. ONE AIDS DEATH EVERY HALF HOUR–a statement that has unfortunately remained true, so the graphic is still in use by AIDS activists.

The success of SEIZE CONTROL OF THE FDA can perhaps best be measured by what ensued in the year following the action. Government agencies dealing with AIDS, particularly the FDA and NIH, began to listen to us, to include us in decision-making, even to ask for our input. Six months prior to SEIZE CONTROL OF THE FDA, members of ACT UP's Treatment and Data Committee had forwarded a detailed critique of the AIDS Clinical Trials Group (ACTG–a reorganized version of the former ATEU system) to the National Institutes of Health. The critique called for a system of parallel trials for experimental AIDS therapies that would allow people excluded from clinical trials to receive the drugs after Phase I studies had been completed. Following the FDA action, ACT UP continued to lobby for parallel trials, meeting with NIH and FDA officials, negotiating with pharmaceutical companies, and testifying before congressional committees. One year after SEIZE CONTROL, ACT UP's idea, now called Parallel Track, was accepted by the NIH and FDA and went into effect for ddI (dideoxyinosine), the first antiviral AIDS drug to become available since AZT.

We Die, They Do Nothing,
1988,
dan keith williams.
Poster, offset lithography,
22 × 17"
(also used as T-shirt).

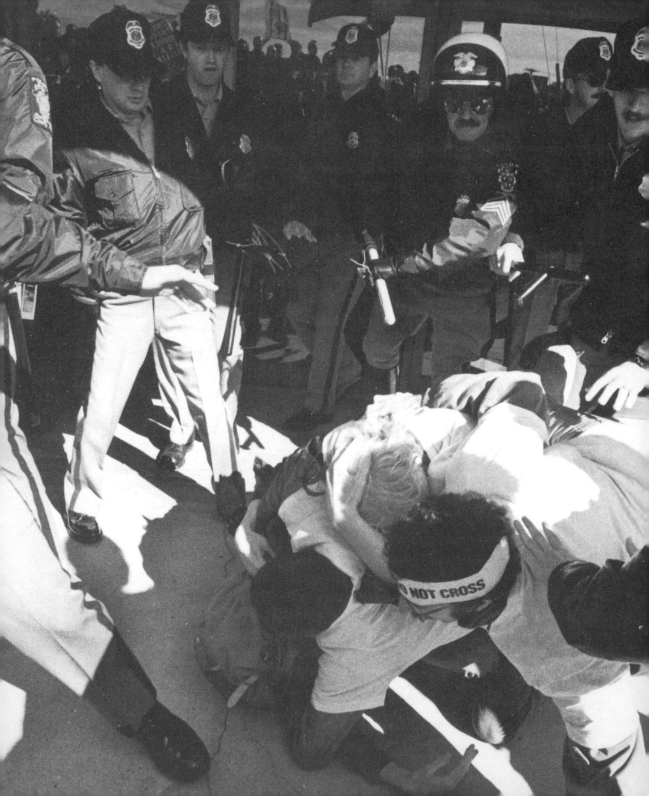

City Hall, New York City, March 28, 1989

Two years after our first demonstration, ACT UP New York decided to target City Hall instead of returning to Wall Street for a third time. Most of ACT UP's major demonstrations had addressed national AIDS issues, in spite of the fact that we live in the city with the largest number of reported cases (nearly 19,000 as of March 1988, 22 percent of the national total) and with one of the worst records in combatting the epidemic. Although we had staged numerous small actions and zaps challenging particular aspects of the Koch administration's negligent AIDS policies, we had not yet focused on New York City's overall scandalous handling of the health crisis. Attention shifted not simply from national to local issues, however, but, more important, from an emphasis on "drugs into bodies"–research funding, the drug approval process, access to treatment–to an emphasis on a wider range of social problems directly intersecting with the epidemic. Many of these problems are the immediate responsibility of city government, no matter how regularly Mayor Koch tried to pass the buck to Albany or Washington, D.C.

The success of SEIZE CONTROL OF THE FDA had taught us much about organizing a major demonstration: the necessity to educate the entire movement about complex issues, the value of an all-out media effort, and the strategic advantage of affinity group tactics. We wanted to add one more dimension to our siege of City Hall: sheer numbers. In addition to massive civil disobedience, we sought participation in a legal picket by thousands of people who had never before joined us in a demonstration. Our outreach efforts were therefore redoubled. We published a special issue of our ACT UP REPORTS newspaper, wheatpasted and handed out fliers for weeks in advance of the demo, even paid for full-page ads in local newspapers. And this time, the media was working for us in advance. For several months in the winter of 1988–89, a constant story in the daily newspapers and on local TV newscasts was the imminent collapse of New York City's health care system. Hospital beds were in short supply; waits of days and even weeks for a bed were the norm–even for those who could afford the price. Emergency rooms were overflowing, partially because of drugs, partially because of AIDS, but more crucially because the city's rapidly increasing poor population has no primary health care and is thus

Photo: Ben Thornberry

forced to resort to public hospital emergency facilities when a doctor is needed. And there were huge shortages of hospital supplies and staff, especially nurses and social workers.

What ACT UP knew, through excruciating experience and diligent research, was that the city's health care crisis was no temporary problem. Rather it was ongoing and systemic, rooted in entrenched social structures and government policies. While social inequities and bad government had grown worse under Mayor Koch's long and tyrannical regime, he had maintained his popularity by appealing to people's worst fears and prejudices. The tide was turning, however, and one small measure of that fact was that Koch seldom asked anymore his famous self-aggrandizing question: "How'm I doin'?" So ACT UP devised a new graphic to sneak into subway-car advertising slots. Beside a picture of a sinister-looking Koch was the text: 10,000 NEW YORK CITY AIDS DEATHS. HOW'M I DOIN'?

In the two weeks prior to TARGET CITY HALL, ACT UP conducted three teach-ins for its own membership and others recruited to the cause. Information from the four-hour sessions was condensed and distributed in TARGET CITY HALL: AN AIDS ACTIVIST'S GUIDE TO NEW YORK CITY IN 1989. Introductory texts in this handbook explain the necessary redefinition of AIDS as symptomatic HIV-related disease (which would qualify people from the entire spectrum of HIV-related illnesses for services), the redefinition of risk as based on behavior instead of identity, and the current epidemiology of AIDS in New York. Next, under the heading WHO'S NOT DOING WHAT, is an outline of the power structure of New York City government and the bureaucratic system of service agencies responsible for various problems directly or indirectly related to AIDS: the Department of Health, Health and Hospitals Corporation, Human Resources Administration, Board of Education, Department of Housing Preservation and Development, and so forth. The bulk of the handbook consists of separate chapters about New York's crises in health care, homelessness, discrimination, drug use, and education; and about various groups affected by AIDS: people of color, women, children and adolescents, gay men and lesbians, sex workers and prisoners. The 100-page book presents a daunting array of problems seemingly requiring vast expenditures to rectify. But as the introduction points out:

Invest in Marble and
Granite,
1989,
Ken Woodard.
Newspaper advertisement,
web offset,
21 × 14½".

WHAT DOES KOCH PLAN TO DO ABOUT AIDS?
INVEST IN MARBLE AND GRANITE.

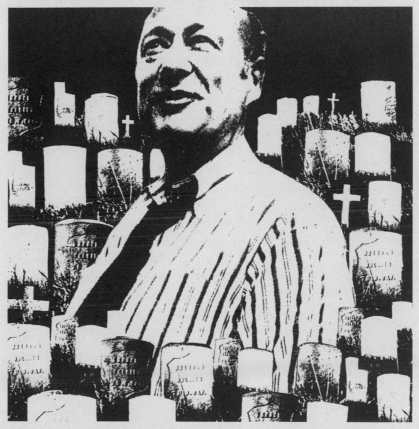

Welcome to New York, where AIDS is good for undertakers but bad for people. About 10,000 people. People the city left to die. And more will die, unless you do something. But what's something you can do?

Simple. Be at City Hall on March 28th at 7:30 a.m. Be a part of the largest AIDS demonstration ever. And what, exactly, are we demonstrating against? A city that spends only one half of one percent of its budget on AIDS. A city whose health department cuts costs by cutting estimates of people infected with HIV. A city where I.V. drug users with AIDS wait ten months to get into a treatment program when, on average, they have six months to live. A city that owns thousands of empty apartments while 5,000 people with AIDS live on the streets. And if you think AIDS only affects the people that get it, think about trying to get a hospital bed when many hospitals in New York are at 95% capacity.

Which is why we're targeting City Hall. And why we're protesting two ways: With a legal picket, and more forcefully, through civil disobedience. Civil disobedience training will be held on March 25th from 12-6 p.m. at The Center, 208 West 13th St. between 7th and 8th Aves.

But whether you want to get arrested or not, join us on the east side of City Hall on March 28th. And if you want to know more about AIDS in NYC before the 28th, come to a teach-in at The Center on March 23rd (7-10 p.m.) or March 26th (3-6 p.m.). It's time we told City Hall to tackle the AIDS crisis, instead of burying it.

AIDS Coalition to Unleash Power, 496 Hudson St. Suite G4, New York, NY 10014 (212) 533-8888.

• Our goals are attainable. Our goals are affordable. Remember, the entire amount requested for 1989 by the Committee for AIDS Funding (a consortium of community-based AIDS groups) is $41 million–just one-sixth of the tax rebate the city gave Chase Manhattan Bank for relocating to Brooklyn instead of New Jersey.

• Remember, New York City is wasting millions on welfare hotels and acute-care beds filled with homeless people who would survive and thrive much better in good old-fashioned apartments–at a fraction of the cost. The same is true of drug treatment versus drug enforcement, and so on and on.

• What we are pressing for–a compassionate continuum of health care, including explicit education, early intervention with known, existing, available drugs, vastly expanded outpatient care, more acute-care beds with more doctors, nurses, and staff; more clinics and drug de-tox programs, addiction treatment on demand; housing options ranging from rent subsidies to supported residences when necessary–these things sound wildly expensive, but they are attainable and, if attained, will save hundreds of millions in hospitalization costs and more hundreds of millions in law enforcement costs, keep people relatively healthy and productive for years if not decades, and make New York once more a livable city.

Information distilled from the TARGET CITY HALL handbook was distributed in three other forms: in press kits with "backgrounders" on

Target City Hall,
1989,
Ken Woodard.
Crack-and-peel sticker,
offset lithography,
6 × 2"
(logo also used for
press kit cover).

Police arrest an ACT UP
member for civil disobedience
at City Hall, New York
City, March 28, 1989 (photo:
Tom McKitterick).

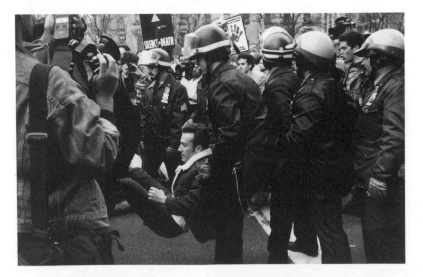

ACT UP
FIGHT
BACK
FIGHT
AIDS
MARCH
28TH
7:30 AM

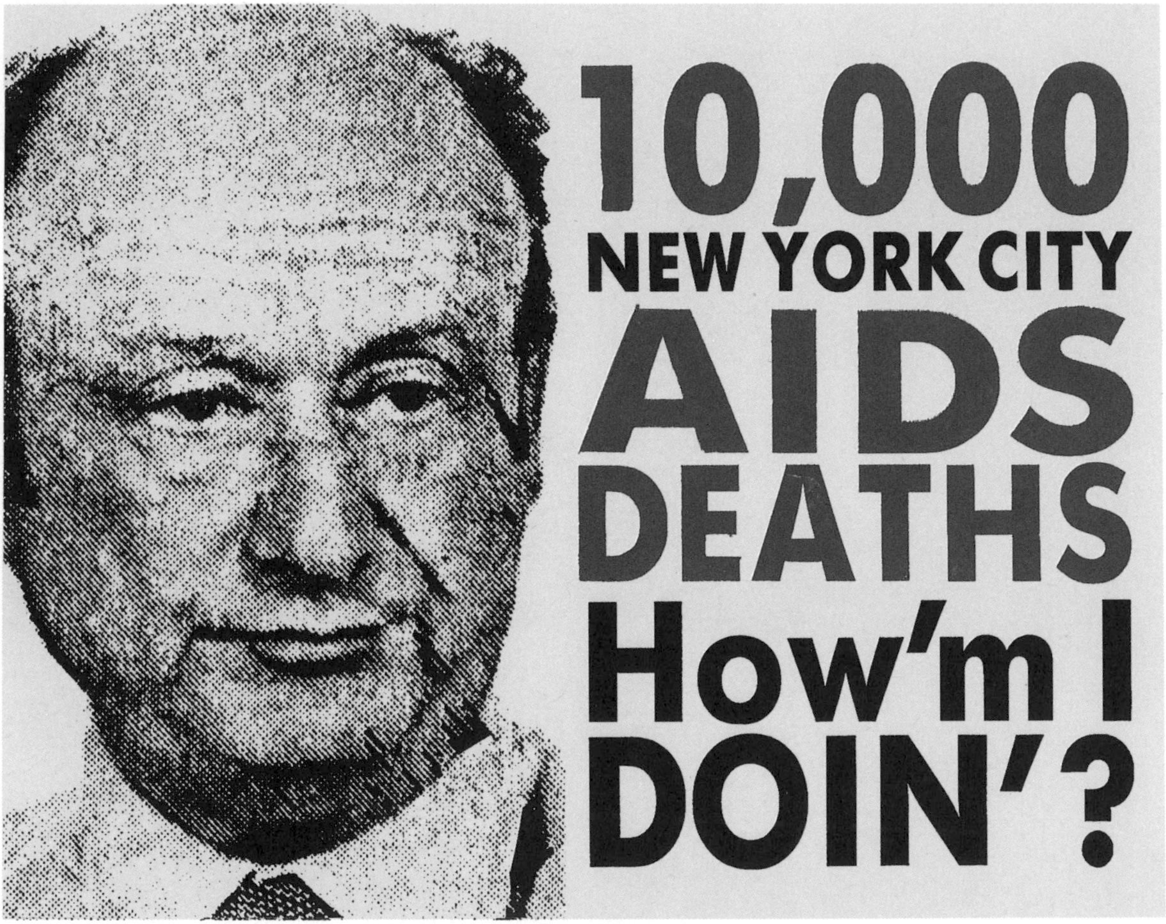

10,000
NEW YORK CITY
AIDS
DEATHS
How'm I
DOIN'?

specific problems, on 12 different REASONS-TO-ACT-UP posters wheat-pasted prior to the demonstration, and on fliers to be handed out at the protest. These are just a few of the points from the flier:

HOSPITALS

FACTS:

• The Health and Hospitals Corporation (HHC) runs 12 city-owned hospitals, which are taking care of 37 percent of New York City's AIDS caseload.

• Koch is cutting the city's contribution to HHC's budget by 8 percent.

• In city hospital emergency rooms, patients must endure four-hour to four-day waits for care.

THE CITY MUST:

• Aggressively fund and support HHC and its municipal hospitals.

• Increase emergency room staff and funding in city hospitals.

• Advocate full state and federal reimbursement for health care in both private and municipal hospitals.

THE HOMELESS

FACTS:

• Partnership for the Homeless estimates that 5,000 city residents with AIDS do not have housing.

• The city provides only 62 beds for homeless people with AIDS.

THE CITY MUST:

• Provide housing–not beds in shelters–to all homeless New Yorkers with AIDS.

• Convert unoccupied city-owned buildings into housing for the homeless and care facilities for homeless people with symptomatic HIV infection.

DRUG USE AND AIDS

FACTS:

• Up to 60 percent of the city's 200,000 IV drug users are estimated to be infected with HIV.

• Only 40,000 openings are available in drug abuse treatment programs. The average wait to get into a program is ten months.

How'm I Doin'?,
1989,
Richard Deagle.
Subway advertising poster,
silk screen,
11 × 13⅞"
(also used as placard).

Reasons to ACT UP
(12 variations),
1989,
Ken Woodard.
Poster, offset lithography,
17 × 11".

REASON #5 TO **ACT UP** ON MARCH 28TH
7:30AM PROTEST AT CITY HALL. CALL ACT UP
AT 212-533-8888 FOR MORE INFO. *TARGET CITY HALL*
ACT UP. THERE'S NO REASON NOT TO.

SINCE THE CITY CUT AIDS EDUCATION, MORE KIDS GET TO LEAVE SCHOOL EARLY.

REASON #12 TO **ACT UP** ON MARCH 28TH

7:30AM PROTEST AT CITY HALL. CALL ACT UP

AT 212-533-8888 FOR MORE INFO.

ACT UP. THERE'S NO REASON NOT TO.

TARGET CITY HALL

FOR MANY BLACKS AND LATINOS UNABLE TO AFFORD AIDS CARE THE COST OF LIVING IS TOO HIGH.

- The city stopped running drug addiction treatment programs during the mid-1970s fiscal crisis, leaving the burden to the state.

THE CITY MUST:

- Resume its role in funding and providing drug abuse treatment programs and ensure that treatment on demand is available to all drug users.

- Provide intensive preventive education and frontline health care services for drug users.

ACT UP's leafleting and wheatpasting, teach-ins and civil disobedience trainings, and its concerted media campaign had the desired effect. At 7 A.M. Tuesday morning, March 28, 5,000 people gathered at City Hall. For the next several hours, as the crowds marched and chanted, wave after wave of affinity groups blocked traffic coming off the Brooklyn Bridge, down Broadway and Chambers Street. The police arrested over 200 protesters, but were largely restrained from the brutality they'd exercised the year before by the presence of hundreds of media people, including our own. (With no cameras around, however, the police illegally strip-searched the women arrestees, hoping the humiliation would deter their further civil disobedience.) Among other preparations for TARGET CITY HALL, video-makers in ACT UP formed a collective called DIVA TV (Damned Interfering Video Activist Television), one member of which was attached to each affinity group to document its activities and provide countersurveillance on the police. DIVA members carried professional-looking press passes of their own making that stated:

- This card identifies the person named on the reverse as an authorized representative of DIVA TV. Please extend to her/him all of the professional privileges and assistance normally extended to the press.

- DIVA TV is an affinity group within ACT UP. We are committed to making media that directly counters and interferes with dominant media assumptions about AIDS and governmental negligence in dealing with the AIDS crisis.

- We are committed to challenging a racist, sexist, and heterosexist dominant media that is complicit with our repressive government.

Gran Fury also provided a bit of their own media in the form of the *New York Crimes*. Designed to resemble the *New York Times*, the four-page

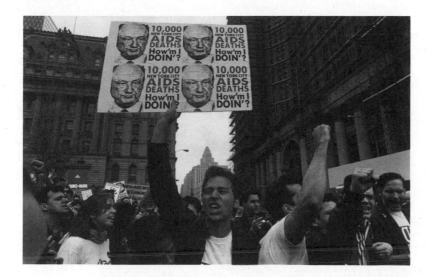

ACT UP demonstration at City Hall, New York City, March 28, 1988 (photo: Ben Thornberry).

New York Crimes,
1989,
Gran Fury.
Four-page newspaper, web offset, each page 22¾ × 15".

newspaper carried stories by ACT UP members on city AIDS issues and graphics by Gran Fury. Beginning at 4 A.M. before the demonstration, Gran Fury members prowled the city, opening *Times* vending boxes and diligently wrapping each newspaper with the *Crimes*. The morning of TARGET CITY HALL, you had—for once—the chance of reading some truth about AIDS in your morning newspaper. And though there was more accurate AIDS reporting in the four-page *Crimes* than has appeared cumulatively in nine years of the *Times*, ACT UP's agenda did come across loud and clear in the media coverage of our biggest and most successful demonstration yet. Apparently Ed Koch wasn't doin' so well. Six months later he would lose the Democratic primary election to the man who became New York City's first Black mayor, David Dinkins.

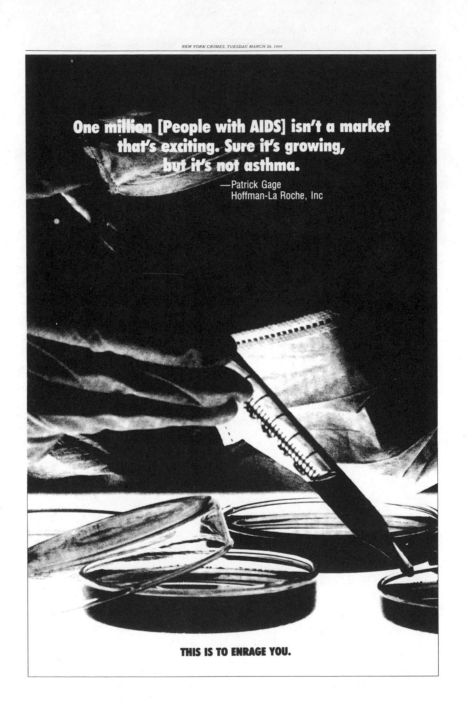

"Men: Use Condoms Or Beat It"

The New York Crimes

Early Edition

New York: Today, high pressure systems likely as storms build and waves break. Highs and lows. Some clouds before completely clearing. Details at City Hall.

NOT TO BE CONFUSED WITH THE NEW YORK TIMES   NEW YORK, TUESDAY, MARCH 28, 1989   FREE

AIDS and Money:

Healthcare or Wealthcare?

Decisions Made Disregard the Sick

Profiteering from healthcare is not news in this country, but AIDS, which stands at the crossroads of medicine, morality and free enterprise, throws the trauma of human greed into sharp focus. The relationship between money and government programs to end the AIDS crisis needs very close scrutiny.

EXAMPLE: AIDS is not yet big enough to be matured by the full attention of the financial community. According to a spokesperson for Hoffman-LaRoche Inc, "there one million AIDS cases is an exciting market, but it's not uniform." Profit incentives come first, even in matters of life and death. Investors place Roche the client, wondering if they will win the big bucks in the race between the development of new drugs and the "short" life expectancy of the people who need them.

EXAMPLE: The complex and rapid FDA protocols for approval of new AIDS drugs works within the constraints of the old line Network AZT, a drug originally invented by the NIH, was sped through the process, while many applications by less competent researchers have been turned for vocational reasons. The FDA office is unreliable to slahealers for permitting their inscrutable systems. Consequently, smaller thysevesiontirely cannot satisfy the impenetrable pro-requisites, stockholders lose faith, and bankruptcy looms. Promising AIDS therapies are lost in the process.

EXAMPLE: Federal spending for AIDS education programs should have only the approval of the few Senate AIDS. However, in an attempt to stop ALL Americans (they are, after all, paying for it) the content of the campaigns is watered down in subcommittees, extracted is all the specific information which is necessary and useful to the affected communities — how to have safe sex and clean needles. The result: AIDS continues to spread, money is wasted, and the individuals that need the information most are walled out.

EXAMPLE: AIDS is consistently compared to other illnesses. Cancer experts state that considering the death toll, the amount of money spent on AIDS is proportionate to the amount spent on cancer. Cancer is not communicable. Nor are cancer patients victimized by discrimination, which can lead to the loss of housing and employment. Some also contend that AIDS is the result of "lifestyle", so it should be the burden of those who are stricken. That is exactly what people said about cancer thirty years ago.

EXAMPLE: Government short cuts, like the call for widespread mandatory testing, fit comfortably with the conservative agenda because they are faster a seemingly concrete result for the money spent. Mandatory testing is pointless, arbitrary segregation. The money remaining issues, from housing to hospitalization to the depletion of this national work force, are ignored. In its myopia, it temporarily lulls the "safe" into feeling safer, and avoids the inescapable long range costs.

So, the next time you pass a noisy demonstration calling for more money to fight AIDS, consider people with AIDS who are being tossed around like political footballs while the powers that be bicker over who will reap the profits from their illness and who will foot the bill for their deaths.

THOUSANDS OF NEW YORKERS MAY BE DYING IN THE STREETS

STATE'S HIGHEST COURT FINDS CITY LEGALLY RESONSIBLE

NEW YORK, Mar 27 — Recently released estimates show that thousands of New Yorkers may die in the streets in the next five years, victims of the Koch administration's callous indifference to homeless people with AIDS.

In another recent development, the New York State Supreme Court reviewed a case that centered around the city's responsibility to provide appropriate housing for a homeless man with AIDS-related complex. In the case, Phillips v Grinder, the court found that the state's Human Resource Administration has a legal responsibility to provide the plaintiff with a separate room rather than a shelter bed, where he would be continually exposed to potentially fatal infections.

Experts claim that City Hall's recently revealed plan to provide 840 beds over the next three years for homeless people with AIDS-PWAs fall drastically — if not criminally — short of what will be needed. Current figures released by the Coalition for the Homeless put the number of PWAs presently living on the street at 8,000. The Coalition, which unlike the city has attempted to verify the size of the homeless PWA population, predicts that by 2001 there will be upwards of 45,000 people with AIDS or HIV infection without homes. If the city meets its own deadlines, the projected facilities — eight sites scattered throughout the Bronx, Brooklyn and Manhattan — will bring to just over 1,000 the total number of beds available, still would still leave over 90 percent of the homeless PWA population living in the streets and shelters, over 44,000 people.

Little Cause for Hope

Ignoring the fact that the city has no plans for the design, development or operation of the facilities — casting doubt on its sincerity of purpose — there is little cause for hope that the city will be able to attain its own pathetically modest goals. The city has so far failed to do two essential promise to build a 72-bed center in Butler House, a 44-bed facility currently the city's only residence for homeless PWAs.

Other factors exist which make it even more unlikely that the city's plans will ever reach fruition. As with the facilities

Continued on next page

WOMEN AND AIDS: OUR GOVERNMENT'S WILLFUL NEGLECT

The AIDS crisis throws the congestion between women and men into sharp relief. When women are dependent on men financially, they are inevitably dependent on them for healthcare. When women are not dependent on men financially, men still control the medical system which provides their care. Women have only recently and partially been included in AIDS studies, the majority of which have been based only on the model of male bodies. These inequities have made it difficult or impossible for women to receive experimental therapies and adequate health care. Women living with AIDS are among the many individuals tied up in the red tape of governmental bureaucracy. Many have died wanting.

AIDS is the leading cause of death for women between the ages of 25-35 in New York City. Of these cases, 51% are Black, 32% are Latino. While women comprise 4% of the national cases, they total 13% of the cases in New York City, and 29% in Newark. 29% of these cases are the result of heterosexual contact, 50% are IV drug users or the sexual partners of IV drug users.

Women are routinely denied access to experimental drug trials. These trials are often the only means of treatment for HIV infected persons. When women are not locked out explicitly by the design of the clinical trials, they are the victims of de facto discrimination; poverty and the lack

Continued on next page

N.Y. HOSPITALS IN RUINS; CITY HALL TO BLAME

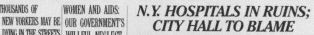

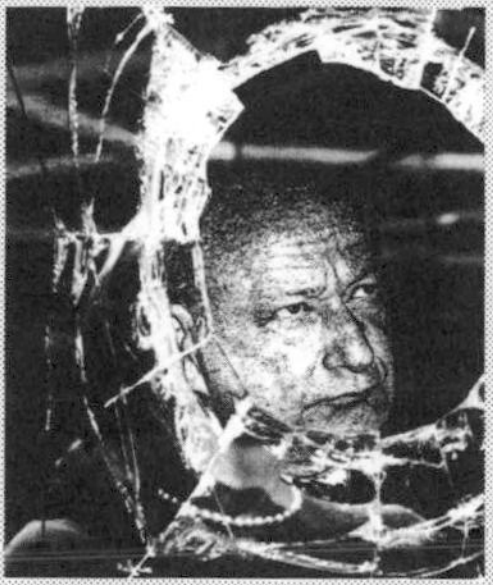

Mayor Koch examines the ruins of New York City after years of his neglect. Critics blame the demise of the hospital system and the lack of AIDS services on his administration.

KOCH FUCKS UP AGAIN

NEW YORK, March 27 — Healthcare in New York City to be the near mayoral candidate dares to address. As the collapse of the city's hospital system appears imminent, most New Yorkers will be affected by the AIDS epidemic that are infected by the human immunodeficiency virus or HIV, the virus believed to cause AIDS.

The city healthcare system, already in severe crisis after more than a decade of inadequate funding, staffing and patient management, must assume a disproportionate share of the burden of AIDS which in this city is increasingly a poor person's disease. Preventive and community medicine for the city poor is virtually nonexistent and the overflow from city hospitals is already threatening to flood the emergency rooms of New York City's voluntary and private hospitals.

The city's "Strategic Plan for AIDS" states that New Yorkers infected with HIV should be treated at local AIDS Accessible Centers. These centers would provide their infected clients with a range of "primary care" services which include monitoring the immune system, treatments for certain medical problems, and preventive therapy against HIV-related opportunistic infections.

"Either inadequate care or none," says a Brooklyn doctor

There are now only two AIDS Assessment centers in the city, both community-based workers complain that this is not nearly enough to treat current need, a need they say grows daily. One of the Centers, the Community Health Program in the Riverside Village section of Manhattan, has a six-month waiting list for new clients. The other Woodhull Clinic in the Bushwick Health Center in Brooklyn, which was treating over 700 people with HIV infection per month in 1988, has stopped taking new patients indefinitely. "This glut means that even people with HIV infection and no health insurance are either receiving no care or going to emergency rooms and receiving inadequate care — or even the wrong care if they're misdiagnosed," said one doctor from the Woodhull Clinic.

The emergency rooms of the public hospitals are asked to provide healthcare to many poor people because primary care facilities in poor communities are overcrowded, inadequate or do not exist, and these emergency rooms are overtaxed in other ways. Although public hospitals have only 16 percent of the acute-care hospital beds in the city, they are caring for more than 35 percent of the people who are hospitalized for AIDS-related conditions in New York City. The resulting shortage of beds means that it is common for patients, with and without AIDS, to wait several days in city emergency rooms until a bed is available.

Empty Beds and No Space

"It would be wrong to think the healthcare crisis results simply from a shortage of facilities," said a leader of a local healthcare workers union. "there's a shortage of staff as well." The public hospitals' freeze on hiring personnel was directly involved in patient care means that the rest of the staff, including nurses and even more doctors, are performing tasks that are essential to a hospital's functioning but unrelated to direct patient care. This, plus the low salaries and the cap on the amount of overtime public hospital personnel can work, all make the prospect of working at a public hospital unattractive. Rumors of these working conditions have exacerbated in New York

Continued on next page

Inmates with AIDS: Inadvertent Political Prisoners

NEW YORK, Mar 27 — A prison is responsible for the health care of its inmates, a responsibility commanded by the Constitution and the Supreme Court. There are currently estimated to be 10,000-20,000 HIV-positive New Yorkers who spent some part of 1988 living as inmates at Rikers Island Prison. Most are distinguished by having a viral which is the leading cause of death among both male and female inmates there. Rikers NYC failed these people in fulfilling that responsibility.

Jose Vasquez thinks so. When he took his first bout with pneumonia in July 1987, he was sent to the Bellevue Hospital prison ward, where a battery of tests were performed, including tests for HIV antibodies and tuberculosis. When his test came back seropositive for HIV, he was returned to Rikers' "AIDS Dorm" where he was housed in the dorms upon ward with 46 other inmates.

Even after he recovered from his pneumonia, and his oral thrush and diarrhea were brought under control, he was not permitted to return to the normal prison population. Prison policy requires that any inmate who has had AIDS-related infection remain in the AIDS Dorm as long as he is held on Rikers. Consequently, Mr Vasquez's compromised immune system was exposed to all the various infections his wardmates

were fighting off.

What he and the other ward residents did not know was that he had an infection. When Bellevue returned the results of his TB test, Mr Vasquez had already been returned to Rikers. Eight months later the TB diagnosis arrived at Rikers. The door blamed, their only made inmates worse. In a classic case of closing the barn door after the horse had escaped, he was placed in an isolation cell after being treated for his TB. The cell's toilet was clogged with feces, papers insulated in and out of broken windows leaving droppings next to his bed, and there was inadequate heat to combat the March cold. He was kept there for two weeks. While there, he was taken off his AZT because he developed a toxic reaction. This is a common problem among people with AIDS with multiple health problems who because of their former drug use and lack of health care. Since AZT is the only drug available to HIV-infected inmates, his immune system continued to deteriorate.

Adequate medical care and non-supported housing are only two of the issues raised by inmates recently incarcerated at Rikers.

Unsafe sex and IV drug use occur on Rikers, but sex and drugs are illegal activities in jail, subjecting prisoners to further punishment. Condoms must be obtained through an infirmary appointment, requiring a kind of advance planning uncharacteristic of sexual behavior among any social group anywhere anytime.

Intravenous drug use was the route of HIV transmission for most of the infected inmates. While most are detained or must go "cold turkey" while at Rikers, no effort is made to bridge their adjustment upon release. Inmate representatives have repeatedly demanded the creation of half-way houses and social services designed to take advantage of one of the few positive aspects of the prison experience — it could save IV drug users' lives. The opportunities are lost when inmates return, homeless and cut off from social services to the streets of New York.

On the other hand, the recent arrest of some Corrections Officers accused of smuggling drugs into the prison system highlights the ostrich-like response of the prison authorities to existing inmate drug use. Corrections officers are the source of the drugs and the handful of needles available — which are used and re-used by the inmates — increasing the likelihood of HIV transmission. The culprit is not only prison guard greed, but lack of adequate education for the inmates. "They give us a couple hundreds and a lecture when we come in, but why you gonna trust when the water people have put thrown you in this hell-hole?" said one inmate. Inmate-initiated peer counselling programs — in their infancy stages in the most conventional system — have not been able to catch hold at Rikers, partly due to population transience. But much more can be done. the interviewed inmates agree.

For Jose Vasquez it has been too little too late. "I pled guilty to attempted robbery, but I didn't know it would be a life sentence," he said. New York State Commission on Correction statistics illustrate the physical distances of AIDS, or treat symptoms of the greater diseases: the terminal conditions of sexism and racism, classism and homophobia.

Continued on next page

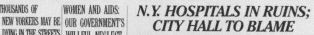

CITY HALL

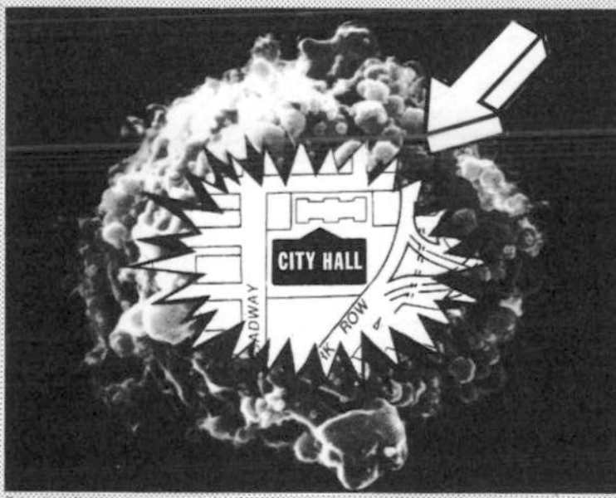

Scientists discover real reason behind the high incidence of HIV infection in New York.

What About People of Color? Race Effects Survival

Studies confirm what people of color have known for a long time: race is a major factor in surviving AIDS. It affects the amount and availability of AIDS information obtainable, and the quality of medical care people receive as well as the financial assistance available to them. It affects societal perceptions of a chronic long term condition.

The face of AIDS has never been totally a white, gay one in this country. The face of this illness is now also the face of a young Latino man or a young African-American woman. The demographics of this disease continue to personalize, as seen by the trail AIDS has cut through the minority communities of this country. As of September 30th, 1987, all reported cases of intravenous drug users with AIDS were people of color. People of color comprise 80 percent of the cases of

heterosexual transmission. Latino and African-American gay men are never married. Of 280 AIDS cases reported to the Minnesota Department of Health, 12 percent of them are people of color. People of color comprise 5.5 percent of Minnesota's population.

Historically, people of color have had limited access to quality healthcare. Consequently, responses to this limited access have developed. In a report published by Harvard medical researchers, we learn that blacks are less likely to have medical insurance than whites. Blacks use emergency rooms and clinics more. They have more difficulty in getting to doctors, hospitals and clinics than whites. Thirty-seven percent of the blacks in this study had not visited a doctor in a year. Of the blacks, 30 percent had not had an annual blood pressure check.

PWAs of color have consistently been denied access to experimental drug trials. A drug trial involving sickle-cell anemia, a disease known to occur almost exclusively in blacks, excluded blacks from the roster.

Nationally, the incidence of AIDS in women of color has risen sharply. Vaginal sex is the primary means of heterosexual transmission. The risk of getting infected after having unprotected sex with the same partner varies from 30 to 45 percent. Negotiation of safer sex techniques for women of color involves battling traditional and religious belief systems; they risk a higher incidence of physical violence and loss of financial support. Among people of color men with AIDS are known to outsurvive women with the disease almost universally.

Children of color make up 78 percent of

the pediatric AIDS cases for children younger than six. Abandoned children of color are the unwilling participants of unethical experimental drug trials, such as the trial at Kings County Medical Center in which children are strapped to hospital beds for a number of hours and are given a harmful placebo, ddI, note: The sterile placebo affects the infant no good and the needle can only be a portal for infection.)

For people of color, the issue is not late healthcare for those with AIDS, but faster healthcare for all, regardless of their sex or sexual preference, skin color or economic situation. In treating the physical diseases of AIDS, we treat symptoms of the greater diseases: the terminal conditions of sexism and racism, classism and homophobia.

INSIDE

Cocaine IV Drug Use Undercounted
Research reveals the projected HIV sero-prevalence amongst IV Drug Users only counts the 250,000 heroin users, ignoring the 600,000 IV cocaine users.

Homeless Teenagers and AIDS
Covenant House, the only New York residence for homeless adolescents, records abstinence to its clients. Meanwhile homeless teenagers often barter sex for food, shelter or money. Covenant House reports 35% of its new clients are HIV positive.

Koch City Plans: AIDS Deaths Help Gentrification
Economic redevelopment could actually benefit from the selective decimation of certain city communities by the AIDS virus. Koch's reasons for redevelopment, realtors' greed and popular homophobia and racism cultivated by his administration, cut a swathe of death throughout the non-heterosexual neighborhoods of western Manhattan, the Lower East Side, south central Queens, central Brooklyn and virtually half of the Bronx.

New York City, June 25, 1989

On the last Sunday in June 1989, the annual gay pride march down Fifth Avenue would take on an added significance. This year we celebrated the 20th anniversary of the Stonewall riot, the opening volley in the formation of the gay liberation movement. ACT UP had participated in the past two years' marches with large, noisy, theatrical contingents, simultaneously angry and celebratory. Though we are a direct-action AIDS activist group, not a gay organization, most of us are lesbian or gay, and all of us are dedicated to fighting homophobia. Indeed, we see ourselves both as direct heirs to the early radical tradition of gay liberation and as rejuvenators of the gay movement, which has in the intervening decades become an assimilationist civil rights lobby.

The entire month of June is now officially recognized by the New York mayor's office as Lesbian and Gay Pride and History Month. Under the auspices of a community group called Heritage of Pride (HOP), various celebratory events are coordinated: an opening ceremony, a rally in Central Park, and the march itself, followed by a festival on Christopher Street and a dance on one of the old Hudson River piers. HOP had arranged for the 1989 kickoff to be an official rechristening of a block-long section of Christopher Street as Stonewall Place. Mayor Koch would make the dedication—and ACT UP would be there to confront him with his inaction on AIDS, which was killing thousands of gay people. We had zapped the mayor at a similar event the year before—a gay history exhibition at the Tweed Courthouse—and had been severely criticized by conservative gay "leaders" for raining on our own community's parade. For us, though, the parade had already been called off by AIDS, and Koch was one of the rainmakers.

Mayor Koch had a dismal record of lukewarm support for our community, and often—as with AIDS—he openly opposed our interests. He was always there, though, when it came to taking credit for our gains, presiding over our celebratory events, joining our marches for a brief moment in front of the TV cameras, always courting our votes. He was the consummate politician, and his hypocrisy was not lost on us. So when he mounted the platform to proclaim the renaming of our street, we held up hastily made tombstones, on which we had written such phrases as KILLED BY

Riot,

1989,

Gran Fury.

Crack-and-peel sticker,

silk screen,

5⅛ × 3½".

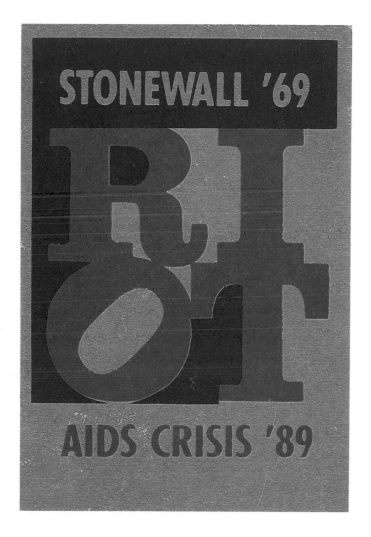

STONEWALL '69

RIOT

AIDS CRISIS '89

KOCH'S INDIFFERENCE; WOMEN DIE TWICE AS FAST; PEOPLE OF COLOR WON'T FORGET THE GENOCIDE. When scores of city cops began pushing us away from the stage, our promised silence gave way to angry shouting, which drowned out the mayor's prepared platitudes. Once more a HOP spokesperson chided *us*, so we drowned her out too. But we were vindicated by the featured speaker of the day, distinguished historian Martin Duberman, who began by saying, "I take no pleasure in sharing a platform with Ed Koch." After praising the kind of people who fought back at Stonewall—drag queens and street people, later scorned by many middle-class gays while reaping the benefits of what they had initiated—Duberman went on to say:

> What we are seeing among the legions of the young who make up ACT UP is once again gay men and lesbian women acting in concert, welcoming and appreciating each other's differentness, and also welcoming minority people. Beyond that change in personnel, what ACT UP has discovered in the process of struggle is the full extent of entrenched privilege which characterizes our society. . . . Because of those insights gathered during ACT UP's struggles, I think we may yet see the birth of a new gay movement which is once more radically oriented.

That was ACT UP's hope, even though most AIDS activists are too young to remember the Gay Liberation Front, to which Duberman compared us. We had chosen IN THE TRADITION: LESBIANS AND GAY MEN FIGHTING BACK for the theme of our participation in the pride celebrations, but we needed to know a little more about that tradition, so a group in ACT UP set about gathering material for another teach-in and handbook—A HIS & HER STORY OF QUEER ACTIVISM.

One piece of our history uncovered by that effort was the symbolism inherent in the route of gay pride marches. In the early 1970s, we had marched out of the gay ghetto, up Sixth Avenue, and into Central Park for a militant rally. We had no police permits; we simply took to the streets and proclaimed our right to be everywhere. By the early 1980s, when we achieved official sanction, the direction was reversed: we walked downtown, into the confines of the gay ghetto, where instead of attending a rally we could drink, eat, dance, and spend our money to enrich Mafia-owned, gay-run businesses. The traditional rally was severed from the march altogether and moved to the preceding day in Central Park. So ACT UP

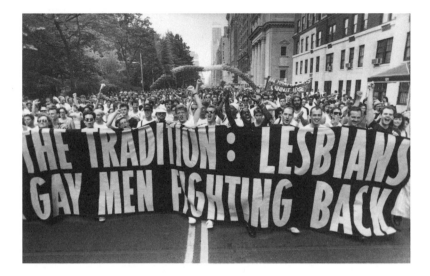

ACT UP and friends march up Sixth Avenue to celebrate the 20th anniversary of the Stonewall riot, New York City, June 24, 1989 (photo: T. L. Litt).

decided to hold a march of our own on Saturday—no police permits, up Sixth Avenue, chanting militantly en route to the rally. By wheatpasting a QUEERS, READ THIS announcement around the city, we got other gay groups to join us, and our ranks swelled to well over a thousand. The police tried to stop us at 14th Street—the dividing line between downtown and uptown—but we were too many, too determined, as we confronted them with our taunting chant:

ARREST US, JUST TRY IT
REMEMBER, STONEWALL WAS A RIOT

As we progressed uptown, we handed thousands of bystanders fliers declaring WHY WE MARCH:

- NOW we march to make history again. WHY NOW?

- NOW we march to fight for our lives!
  Since 1980, 11,200 people in New York City have died from HIV disease. It was the homophobia of the Reagan government and the medical establishment that labeled AIDS a "gay disease" and left us and others to die. It is the homophobia, racism, and sexism of the Koch administration that lowers the estimate of AIDS cases in New York City to save money instead of lives.

- NOW we march to continue to fight against and to expose the connections between homophobia, misogyny, and racism.

We march to eliminate sodomy laws that exist in 25 states, laws that not only invalidate our lives but prevent us from seeking health care for fear of repression. We must all come out against a Supreme Court that not only denies lesbians and gay men the freedom to engage in consensual sex but also is eroding every day the civil rights that protect all minorities. We march in solidarity with others and will not allow one community to be pitted against another.

● NOW we march to demand self-determination.
We have been denied our rights to care for our sick lovers and friends, have lost our housing because our relationships are not considered legitimate, and have had our children taken from us because we are not considered to be fit parents. As women loving women and men loving men, we march together to affirm our love for one another, our dignity and self-worth. We march to demand the recognition of our relationships, for self-determination in matters of health care, housing, and social services, and to keep our children and to become adoptive parents.

● NOW we march to take our lives into our own hands. We march for our liberation.

● RIGHTS ARE GIVEN, LIBERATION IS TAKEN! COME OUT, WAY OUT!

I Am Out,
Therefore I Am,
1989,
Adam Rolston.
Crack-and-peel sticker,
offset lithography,
3⅛ × 3⅛"
(also used as T-shirt).

Coming out of the closet, declaring oneself to the world as gay or lesbian, has been one of the gay movement's sacred tenets, the central act of identity politics. For the 20th anniversary of Stonewall the statement was given a new graphic emblem, ACT UP's T-shirt with an image appropriated from artist Barbara Kruger. Rewriting Descartes's cogito, Kruger took a swipe at consumer-determined identity: I SHOP, THEREFORE I AM. Our graphic played a Foucauldian twist on hers, turning the confession of sexual identity into a declaration of sexual politics: I AM OUT, THEREFORE I AM.

The complex levels of reference in I AM OUT were true of another graphic emblem made for Stonewall 20, Gran Fury's RIOT. The linkage of STONEWALL '69 and AIDS CRISIS '89 by the exhortation to RIOT fit precisely with ACT UP's IN THE TRADITION theme. But the origin of the image is more complicated. Gran Fury had been invited to participate in an art exhibition about AIDS in Berlin the preceding December, and the group wanted to comment on the show's inclusion of the art world's best-known graphic work about AIDS—General Idea's appropriation of Robert Indiana's famous pop art LOVE logo. The Canadian art collective's square

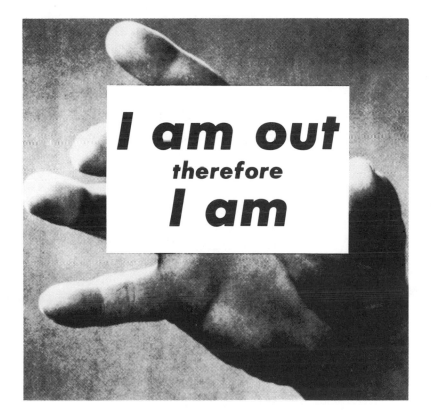

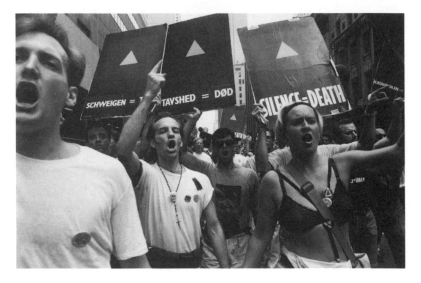

ACT UP members show that silence = death in any language during the gay pride march, New York City, June 25, 1989 (photo: Ellen B. Neipris).

AIDS paintings, posters, and stickers exhibited their usual cynical detachment. What can the word AIDS mean in this format? Did sixties' love lead inexorably to eighties' AIDS? So Gran Fury contributed a six-by-six-foot hard-edge painting of RIOT, using the red, black, and gold of the German flag, an image easily reworked for the celebration of the most famous riot in gay liberation history.

ACT UP's participation in the Sunday pride march was bigger than ever in 1989, and it put AIDS squarely on the march's agenda. Behind three huge banners asking IF NOT NOW, WHEN?, IF NOT HERE, WHERE?, IF NOT US, WHO?, scores of activists carried graphics with statistical information about time and place (*we* were the "who"):

- U.S., JUNE 1989, 39,180 LIVING WITH AIDS, 55,000 DEATHS, 1.5 MILLION HIV-POSITIVE.

- ONE U.S. AIDS DEATH EVERY 30 MINUTES.

- REAGAN: 8 YEARS, NOTHING DONE. BUSH: 157 DAYS AND COUNTING.

- NYC AIDS CARE: PWAS GET LITTLE, PWARCS GET LESS, HIV+ GET NONE.

- IN NYC, BLACKS AND LATINOS = 84% OF WOMEN WITH AIDS, 91% OF INFANTS WITH AIDS, 39% OF GAY MEN WITH AIDS.

● NYC TREATMENT FOR DRUG USERS: NOTHING AT ALL FOR 4 OUT OF 5, COME BACK IN 6 MONTHS FOR 1 OUT OF 5.

The weekend following gay pride day is the Fourth of July, whose celebration in 1989 rang particularly hollow. The U.S. Supreme Court–notorious to us for its decision three years earlier in *Bowers v. Hardwick* to uphold state antisodomy laws–had just handed down a number of decisions severely limiting the possibility of legal redress for civil rights violations. And the further restriction of a woman's right to choose an abortion came from the Reagan court on July 3 in *Webster v. Reproductive Health Services*. At the same time, the Court's decision that desecration of the American flag is legal under the First Amendment was being used by the Right to whip the nation into a furor of purely symbolic patriotism.

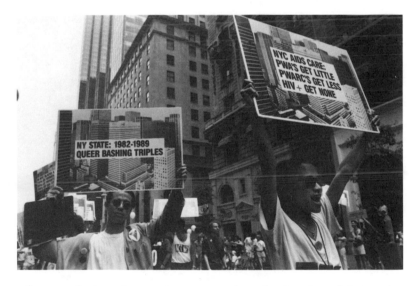

ACT UP members carry placards behind a banner asking "If not here, where?" in the gay pride march, New York City, June 25, 1989 (photo: Ellen B. Neipris).

The contradiction of expressing outrage about flag burning while remaining silent about the abrogation of rights for which the flag supposedly stands was apparently lost on politicians and pundits. Not on ACT UP. We produced a guerrilla subway poster to make the point and arranged our own little flag-burning ceremony in Sheridan Square. Meanwhile, skin heads rampaged through the city beating up anyone speaking out for civil rights; city police sided with the neofascists and arrested dissenters.

AIDS Facts,
(24 variations),
1989,
ACT UP ad hoc
Gay Pride Committee.
Placard, velox,
30 × 40".

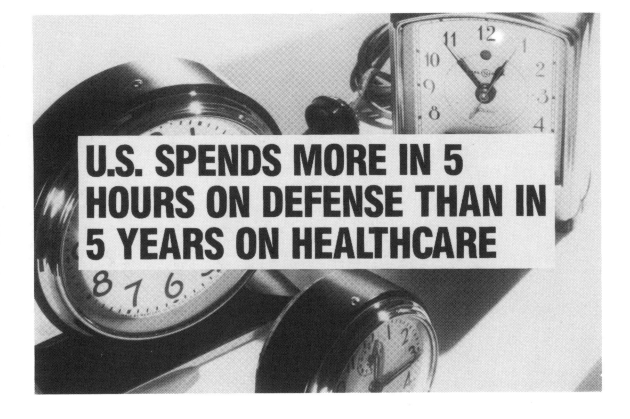

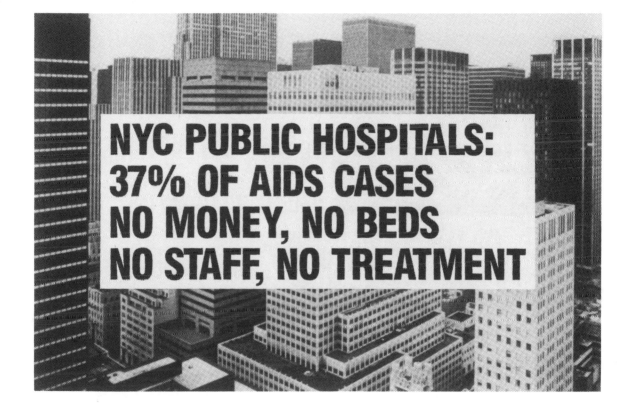

NYC PUBLIC HOSPITALS:
37% OF AIDS CASES
NO MONEY, NO BEDS
NO STAFF, NO TREATMENT

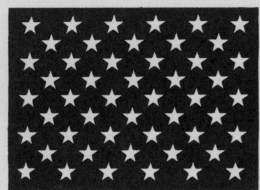 **OUR GOVERNMENT CONTINUES TO IGNORE THE LIVES, DEATHS AND SUFFERING OF PEOPLE WITH HIV INFECTION BECAUSE THEY ARE GAY, BLACK, HISPANIC OR POOR. BY JULY 4, 1989 OVER 55 THOUSAND WILL BE DEAD. TAKE DIRECT ACTION NOW. FIGHT BACK. FIGHT AIDS.**

"Punch" Sulzberger's Fifth Avenue residence and the New York Times Company, New York City, July 26, 1989

A book will one day be written about the *New York Times*'s continuous failure to report the AIDS crisis accurately—if at all. It will no doubt begin with the infamous comparison noticed by Larry Kramer:

- During the first 19 months of the AIDS epidemic (by the end of which time there had been 891 reported cases), the *Times* carried **s e v e n** articles about it, **n o n e** of them on the front page.

- During the three months of the Tylenol scare in 1982 (seven cases), the *Times* carried **f i f t y - f o u r** articles about it, **f o u r** of them on the front page.

If all along, the failure of official policymakers to respond to the epidemic was a result of their disregard for the populations in which the disease was first noticed—primarily gay men—the *New York Times* seconded their contempt. Homophobia is notorious at the *Times*, well known by any lesbian or gay man who reads the paper and every day sees news about us distorted, trivialized, or completely ignored; known, too, from stories told by closeted gay people working on the inside—closeted because being openly gay at the *Times* is cause for immediate dismissal. It took **e i g h t e e n** years of pressure from lesbian and gay organizations to get the *Times* to use the word *gay* instead of *homosexual*, and the paper does so now reluctantly and selectively. When AIDS began to claim the lives of more and more gay men, the *Times* adamantly refused to report AIDS as the cause of death or to list gay lovers among surviving family members. And the *Times* insists on "AIDS victims" against the express wishes of people with AIDS, who prefer precisely that: people with AIDS.

But those of us in the AIDS activist movement know the depth of the *Times*'s contempt to be far greater. Because of the newspaper's racism, sexism, and class bias, **n o o n e** affected by AIDS appears to matter to *Times* editors and writers, or to be understood as included among their readers—no one, that is, but the "exceptional" "victims": the white middle-class hemophiliac child, the white middle-class heterosexual transfusion recipient. Because **w e** don't count for the *Times*, AIDS has been a minor news story, one that doesn't require full-time specialized reporters, investigative reporters, reporters knowledgeable of the science and politics of

American Flag,
1989,
Richard Deagle,
Tom Starace,
and Joe Wollin.
Subway advertising poster,
silk screen,
11 × 14⅝"
(also used as T-shirt).

AIDS. The *New York Times* sent **o n e** reporter to the Fifth International AIDS Conference in Montreal, attended by over 12,000 people (*New York Newsday*, a tabloid, sent **f i v e**). The *Times* reporter didn't bother to attend the opening ceremonies, which were commandeered by hundreds of international AIDS activists in order to read a MANIFESTO OF THE RIGHTS OF PEOPLE WITH AIDS—just one more AIDS story the *Times* therefore missed (national network news programs found time for it even though it happened the same day the Ayatollah Khomeini died and hundreds of Chinese students were massacred in Tiananmen Square).

Least of all does the *Times* feel the necessity of having its reporters consult with people with AIDS or people working within the communities most seriously affected by the epidemic. One *Times* reporter confessed, "*Times* editors discourage use of the word *community;* they consider it jargon." The most serious result of the *Times*'s failure to imagine those of us living every day with AIDS as among its readership is its failure to cover drug treatment and access issues. ACT UP's expertise in these areas has made us all the more painfully aware of the *Times*'s blind prejudice, its ignorance, and its disinterest in saving lives.

ACT UP considered going after the *Times* on several occasions, but always opted for less intransigent adversaries or those whose ignorance or arrogance might be modified by public pressure. But a *Times* editorial of June 29, 1989, titled "Why Make AIDS Worse Than It Is?" was the last straw. In its desire to reassure its readers that the epidemic was leveling off and in any case would never be *their* worry, the editorial typified the newspaper's often-repeated position on AIDS, but this one reached new heights of callousness. The editorial's argument had often appeared before in right-wing journals: that those of us fighting the epidemic, especially the "powerful gay lobby," exaggerate forecasts in order to get more funding (one wonders, do the officially reported 100,000 + cases have to be exaggerated in order to make someone—the *Times*, say—pay attention?). According to the *Times*, dire predictions for the future are misguided. AIDS is "leveling off" because "the disease is still very largely confined to specific risk groups. Once all susceptible members are infected, the numbers of new victims will decline." In other words, "Soon all the fags and junkies will be dead, and we'll be rid of AIDS." The *Times* thus reveals why it still prefers to think about AIDS epidemiology in terms of "risk groups" rather than risk behaviors.

Buy Your Lies Here,
1989,
ACT UP Outreach
Committee.
Crack-and-peel sticker,
offset lithography,
4¼ × 5½".

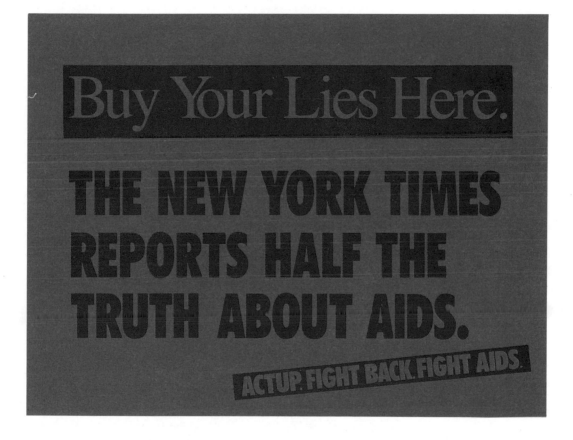

As ACT UP began planning an action, the Outreach Committee struck immediately with two crack-and-peel stickers, BUY YOUR LIES HERE for newsstands and OUT OF ORDER to place over the coin slot of *Times* vending machines. Another recently invented technique was set in motion: a fax zap. The *Times*'s fax numbers were distributed at the weekly meeting, and ACT UP members were encouraged to use our employers' fax machines to jam those at the newspaper with our complaints.

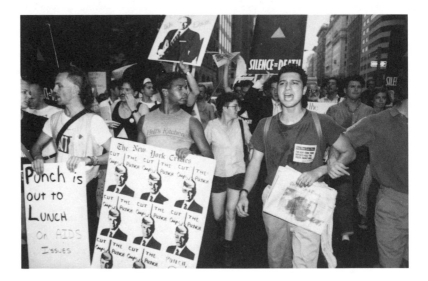

ACT UP demonstrators march down Fifth Avenue on the way from Punch Sulzberger's residence to the New York Times building, New York City, July 26, 1989 (photo: Tom McKitterick).

Out of Order,
1989,
ACT UP Outreach Commitee.
Crack-and-peel sticker, offset lithography, 4¼ × 2¼".

Because *Times* policy is set at the top, ACT UP decided on publisher Arthur "Punch" Sulzberger's Fifth Avenue residence as a starting point for our protest. During the night of July 23, the streets outside Sulzberger's apartment were painted with outlines of bodies and the inscription ALL THE NEWS THAT'S FIT TO KILL. Three days later, 200 ACT UP members gathered at the same spot for an angry demonstration. Fliers with a series of questions were handed out to Punch's neighbors:

- Why does the *Times* refuse to print information about new AIDS treatments until long after their discovery?

- Why, instead of actively investigating the work of federal health organizations, does the *Times* merely rewrite the press releases of the Food and Drug Administration, the Centers for Disease Control, and the National Institutes of Health, among others?

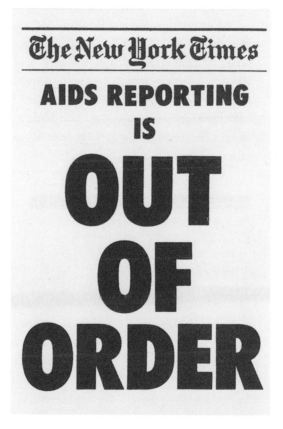

- Why does the *Times* currently have no AIDS reporter in Washington, D.C., the city from which most crucial treatment policies originate?

- Why would the *Times* write an editorial that supports New York City health commissioner Stephen Joseph's plan for an end to anonymous testing and the implementation of contact tracing, a proposal repudiated by both the medical community and a panel of AIDS experts?

At the demonstration, ACT UP found out just how much clout the newspaper has in New York City: the police department guarded Sulzberger's residence with ranks equal in number to our own, and not a single story about the protest appeared in the mainstream media. Deterred at the publisher's digs, ACT UP's legions proceeded to march down Fifth Avenue and over to the *Times* offices on West 43rd Street. There we were met with an even bigger police gang, fully determined to protect the *Times*'s property rights against our own rights of free assembly and speech.

SELL WELLCOME, FREE AZT

New York Stock Exchange, New York City, September 14, 1989

In early September 1989, the government announced the results of a study that showed what informed community physicians and their HIV-positive patients had known for some time: that AZT can delay the onset of disease symptoms. The fact that hundreds of thousands of others with asymptomatic HIV infection would now want the drug resulted in a more than 40 percent increase in the value of shares of Wellcome PLC stock (Wellcome PLC is the British-owned parent company of Burroughs Wellcome, which holds the AZT monopoly). Nevertheless, at a meeting with AIDS activists on September 5, the pharmaceutical company adamantly refused to lower the drug's price.

ACT UP's very first demonstration on Wall Street had decried the exorbitant cost of AZT and the government's refusal to release other promising therapies for AIDS. Now, two and a half years and hundreds of protests later, AZT was still the only licensed antiviral AIDS drug and, at the reduced price of $8,000 per year per patient, still the most expensive drug in pharmaceutical history. Burroughs Wellcome's claim that its huge profit margin was required to offset the drug's development and the fact that it could quickly be replaced by a better drug was growing more specious every day. And the company still refuses to open its books to back up its argument.

AZT was first synthesized as a potential anticancer treatment in 1964 at the Detroit Institute of Cancer Research. The research was supported by a government grant. In 1985 Dr. Samuel Broder of the National Cancer Institute (NCI) discovered AZT's in-vitro effectiveness against HIV. After Burroughs Wellcome completed preclinical trials, the FDA approved AZT as an investigational new drug, and the pharmaceutical company, together with NCI, went on to conduct the first two phases of human trials. In 1986, AZT became a so-called orphan drug for AIDS, followed by the same classification for ARC in 1987. This designation by the FDA grants seven years of tax credits in addition to marketing exclusivity. A use patent granted by the U.S. Patent Office additionally gave Burroughs Wellcome a 17-year exclusive right to manufacture AZT and control its price.

Thus the government subsidized AZT every step of the way—and continues to do so. Most of the postmarketing clinical studies of AZT are funded by the National Institute of Allergy and Infectious Diseases (NIAID). And in 1987 Congress voted a grant program for state governments to pay for AZT for patients who cannot afford it. ACT UP's FDA ACTION HANDBOOK had laid all this out in the fall of 1988. The handbook concluded:

> By colluding with the profiteering of Burroughs Wellcome, the FDA ensured that AZT became a government-sponsored corporate windfall. The federal government paid for the drug's development. The federal NCI confirmed AZT's anti-HIV activity. The federal NIAID AIDS drug trials program is testing new uses for the drug at no cost to the manufacturer. To add to the company's coffers, already bulging with tax credits and a lucrative monopoly, Congress appropriated $30 million to buy the drug for indigent people with AIDS. Thus, the drug, originally developed at federal expense, now soaks up tax dollars to subsidize a secretive, profit-hoarding pharmaceutical monopoly.

On April 25, 1989, an affinity group of four ACT UP members calling themselves the Power Tools walked into the Burroughs Wellcome offices at Research Triangle, North Carolina. Dressed as businessmen, they talked their way past security, went upstairs, and talked a secretary out of her office. They shut the door, opened their briefcases, pulled out their equipment, and sealed themselves in by bolting steel plates to the door frame.

AIDS®
IT'S BIG BUSINESS!
(BUT WHO'S MAKING A KILLING?)

They then called the media, told them who and where they were, and issued their demands that Burroughs Wellcome lower the price of AZT by at least 25 percent and subsidize the cost of the drug for the needy. The police had to break down the office walls in order to arrest the Power Tools. It was one more media strike against Wellcome's profiteering (the *New York Times* missed the story).

On September 14, the reorganized Power Tools struck again. At about 9:25 A.M., seven men dressed as bond traders entered the New York Stock Exchange using faked Bear Stearns name tags. Five of them quickly walked up to the VIP balcony overlooking the trading floor, chained themselves to a bannister, and just as the opening bell went off, dropped a huge banner that said SELL WELLCOME. They then drowned out the traders with the piercing sound of marine foghorns, successfully stopping transactions on the exchange for five minutes–a historical first. The remaining two Power Tools quickly snapped photographs, walked outside, and handed their smuggled-in cameras to waiting ACT UP members, who rushed the pictures to the Associated Press (the *New York Times* missed the story, which appeared on the front page of the *Wall Street Journal*). All seven were arrested and charged with, among other things, criminal impersonation, a class A misdemeanor that ACT UP interpreted as "bad stockbroker drag."

An hour or so after the Power Tools were taken away, 1,500 ACT UP activists arrived at the scene for a demonstration and pandemonium. We too had foghorns, hundreds of them–and earplugs. We also had hundreds of placards and leaflets for the curious lunchtime crowd that gathered, fingers in ears. The leaflet, headed SELL WELLCOME, FREE AZT, outlined the facts of government-sponsored pharmaceutical profiteering on AZT, ending with these:

It's Big Business,
1989,
ACT UP Outreach
Committee.
Subway advertising poster,
offset lithography,
11 × 22"
(also used as placard).

- Wellcome effectively places the drug **o u t   o f   r e a c h** of entire continents such as Africa, where AIDS has reached pandemic proportions. Given Wellcome's large investment in South Africa, THIS IS MEDICAL APARTHEID.

- Locally, Wellcome's profiteering effectively keeps AZT **o u t   o f   r e a c h** of the majority of HIV-infected people: people of color, women, and children.

- THE BOTTOM LINE: We demand that AZT be provided **f r e e - o f - c h a r g e** to all those who wish to use this treatment. With a million and a half Americans infected with HIV and millions more infected worldwide, ANYTHING ELSE WOULD BE GENOCIDE.

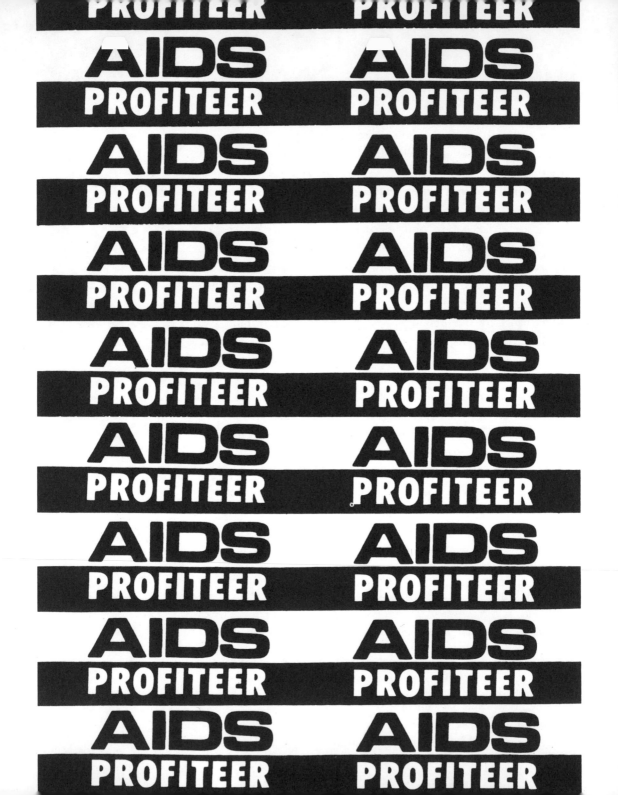

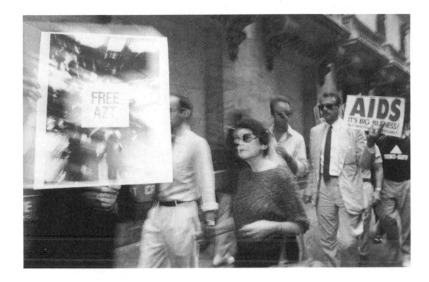

ACT UP demonstration in front of the New York Stock Exchange, New York City, September 14, 1989 (photo: Ben Thornberry

AIDS Profiteer,
1989,
ACT UP Outreach Committee.
Stick-on labels, offset lithography on Avery labels, each label 1 × 2⅞".

ACT UP San Francisco and ACT UP London held demonstrations on the same day, and the following day Wellcome PLC shares fell substantially on the London stock exchange. Four days later Burroughs Wellcome announced a 20 percent reduction in the price of AZT. But at the new price of $1.20 per capsule (Dr. Mathilde Krim of the American Foundation for AIDS Research estimates the production cost of a capsule of AZT to be between 7 and 15 cents), the drug would still cost every patient over $6,000 a year. ACT UP decided to maintain its boycott, announced to the press during the stock exchange demo, of Burroughs Wellcome's over-the-counter drugs. Until AZT is available at no cost to those who need it, AIDS PROFITEER labels will be affixed to packages of Sudafed, Actifed, Neosporin, and other Burroughs Wellcome products at your local drugstore.

Wellcome PLC,
AIDS Profiteer,
1989,
Vincent Gagliostro.
Placard, velox,
24 × 18".

Free AZT,
1989,
Vincent Gagliostro.
Placard, velox,
24 × 18".

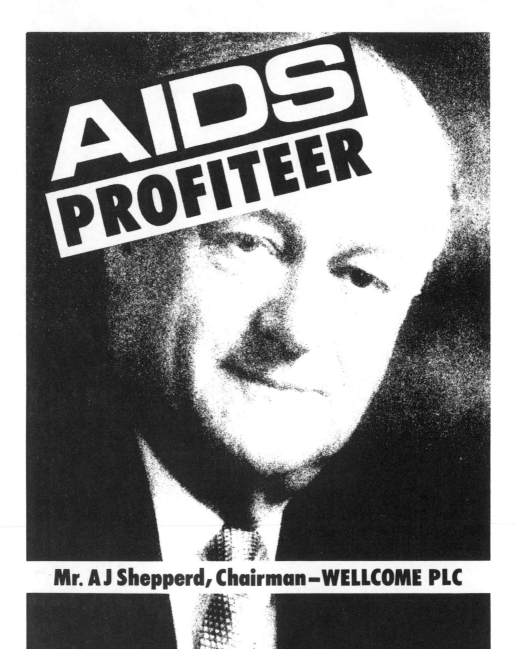

Mr. A J Shepperd, Chairman – WELLCOME PLC

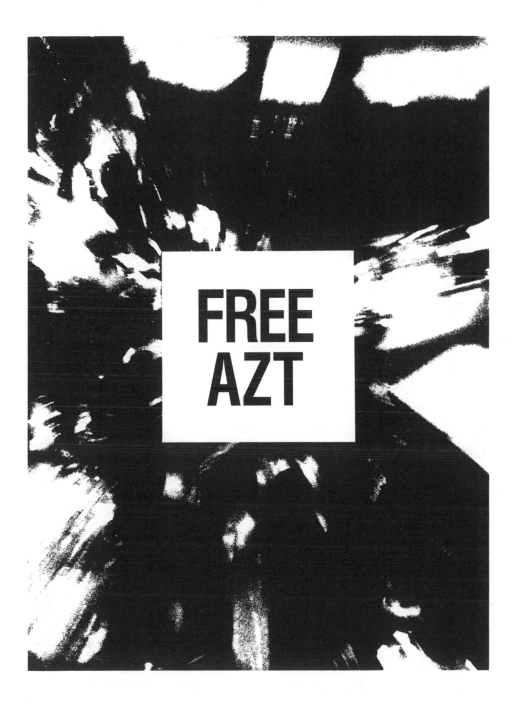

As if having AIDS or being homeless were not horrible enough in itself, imagine the nightmare of being a homeless person with AIDS. This is the condition of an estimated 5,000 to 10,000 New Yorkers. Many more thousands of homeless men, women, and children are HIV-infected. And the city government often won't even acknowledge the problem, much less do anything about it. From the beginning of ACT UP, we knew there were far more homeless people with AIDS (PWAs) in New York than could be housed in the one 44-bed facility that the city provided in 1987 (in response to massive pressure). But we realized the true dimensions of this particular crisis only when we formed the Caucus to House Homeless PWAs (later the PWA Housing Committee) in the fall of 1988. Our first demonstration tackling the issue was scheduled for the day after Thanksgiving 1988, "the biggest shopping day of the year," at Trump Tower. Our reasons for demonstrating at a famous building housing million-dollar apartments and a luxury shopping mall were spelled out in a handout:

- Donald Trump received a tax abatement of $6,208,773 to build Trump Tower. This money could have rehabilitated about 1,200 city-owned apartments. Instead Trump gets richer while homeless people get sicker.

Demand Housing,
1989,
John Consigli.
T-shirt, silk screen,
9½ × 10"
(also used as button).

- The city favors private developers like Trump over small community-based organizations that are committed to providing low-income housing and housing for PWAs. The AIDS Center of Queens County, for example, never even received an acknowledgment of the proposal it submitted for 20 scattered-site apartments for homeless PWAs.

- Mayor Koch and the city allow Trump to displace people from their apartments when he wants to build a building. Trump is symbolic of a system that lets the rich do whatever they want while letting the poor die.

It was a somewhat sketchy presentation of the problem, but by the time of TARGET CITY HALL the following spring, ACT UP's PWA Housing Committee had thoroughly examined both the structural causes of homelessness and the city housing bureaucracy, specifically concentrating on how these affect impoverished people with AIDS. Among the committee's findings were the following: With an estimated 8,000 homeless PWAs in New York

ACT UP

DEMAND HOUSING
FOR HOMELESS PEOPLE
LIVING WITH AIDS

City, the city provides some form of housing for 1,316. Virtually none of it is adequate. Rent subsidies are too low. Single-room-occupancy hotels, where many must live, are run down, unsanitary, ill-heated, and lacking private bathrooms and kitchen facilities. PWAs forced to stay in hospitals are virtual prisoners. And hospitals often refuse to diagnose AIDS because of their legal responsibility not to discharge a PWA onto the street. For those with HIV-related disease and no AIDS diagnosis, the city provides no special housing at all.

The city's much-heralded 1988 plan to provide new housing units for 800 PWAs by 1991 (by which time it is estimated that there will be 30,000 homeless PWAs in New York City) was not only too little too late, but was never seriously intended to be carried out. Koch announced the eight proposed sites to the media without ever having consulted community leaders, thereby ensuring their opposition, especially because he selected locations already overburdened with shelters and drug treatment facilities. Six of the eight buildings were intended to house over 100 PWAs, far too many for such an institution. The death rate at the 44-bed Bailey House is one every 9 to 12 days, which is already unbearable for staff and clients.

Forced to live in shelters and on the streets, PWAs are even more vulnerable to the violence and illnesses that all homeless people face. Homeless people with AIDS are routinely beaten and sometimes killed in shelters, and they are easily exposed to opportunistic infections in filthy, crowded, and disease-ridden facilities. For example, after declining for 15 years, rates of tuberculosis, to which people with impaired immune systems are particularly susceptible, have recently risen sharply. And HIV infection is allowed to spread unchecked in the homeless population, which receives no information about safe sex and needle use, in spite of the fact that as many as 50 percent of the men who live in some shelters have sex with other men, and 20 to 30 percent are IV drug users. Meanwhile, the city has conducted a virtual war against homeless people who avoid shelters, confiscating their belongings and forcibly removing them from parks, the transit system, and public buildings such as train and bus stations.

In a series of protests, zaps, letter-writing campaigns, and meetings in 1989, ACT UP put relentless pressure on New York City's Human Resources Administration (HRA), whose Division of AIDS Services is responsible for providing social services to people with HIV infection, and the Department of Housing Preservation and Development (HPD), which is mandated to work with HRA to develop sites to house homeless PWAS. We demanded:

- That HPD designate ten buildings of at least 20 apartments each out of the over 3,500 vacant buildings managed by HPD to be renovated and used as scattered-site apartments for homeless people with HIV-related illnesses.

- That the city provide the necessary capital funds for the renovation of these buildings.

- That the selection of these buildings be made in collaboration with community leaders and AIDS and housing activists to ensure proper location.

- That from the over 10,000 annually vacated city-owned apartments, HPD and Mayor Koch release and renovate to medically appropriate standards 100 apartments per month (starting June 1989) for homeless people with HIV-related illnesses, symptomatic and asymptomatic, in coordination with HRA services.

Homelessness, including PWA homelessness, extends well beyond New York City, of course. Over 3 million people are homeless nationwide. The federal government's housing policies, especially under the Reagan administration, have directly contributed to the recent precipitous decline in publicly supported and otherwise affordable housing stock in cities throughout the country. In the fall of 1989, homeless people and their advocates organized a mass demonstration in the nation's capital, hoping to make President Bush stick to his campaign promises to solve the housing shortage. The protest was set for Columbus Day weekend, the same weekend that the Names Project quilt would be unfurled on the Ellipse behind the White House. Since then, the quilt has grown too large to be shown in its entirety. Presumably, therefore, no American president will ever see it, since George Bush refused to walk even one city block to pay tribute to those who have died of AIDS. But ACT UP was there, asking others to join us the next day at the HOUSING NOW march to DEMAND HUMANE HOUSING FOR PEOPLE WITH AIDS. Busloads of us had gone down to Washington to be part of the ACT UP AIDS contingent and to network with other housing activists, working to form the coalitions that will be necessary to change a society that treats such basic human needs as housing and health care as privileges, not rights.

ACT UP's message at HOUSING NOW was simple: THE HOUSE THAT JACK BUILDS MUST HOUSE HOMELESS PEOPLE WITH AIDS. Jack Kemp, secretary of

*Humane Housing for
People with AIDS,
(verso),*

*U.S. Gov't Approves
AIDS Ware-Housing
(recto)
1989,
ACT UP PWA Housing
Committee.
Placard, silk screen
on foamcore,
30 × 40".*

HUMANE HOUSING FOR
PEOPLE WITH AIDS.

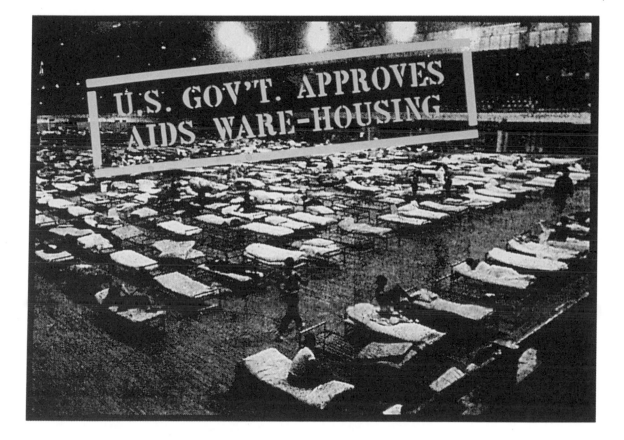

the Department of Housing and Urban Development (HUD), makes the claim that housing *all* homeless people is his number-one priority. But apparently he doesn't know about homeless people with AIDS:

- FACT: Studies estimate that at least 10 percent of all homeless people in the United States are HIV-infected.

- FACT: The incidence of HIV infection is rising fastest among women and people of color. Similarly, the number of homeless women and people of color is increasing faster than any other population.

- FACT: The U.S. government has **n o   p l a n** to house homeless people with AIDS.

- FACT: The McKinney Act, which funds housing for disabled homeless people—named after Stewart McKinney, a congressman who died of AIDS—does **n o t   p r o v i d e** funds for housing people with AIDS.

- FACT: To qualify for housing under the McKinney Act, a homeless person with AIDS must prove that a physical disability existed **b e f o r e** an AIDS diagnosis.

- Once again, the government's response to people with AIDS: LET THEM DIE OFF.

- IT'S TIME TO BRING PRESSURE TO BEAR ON JACK KEMP AND HUD.

ACT UP'S HOUSING NOW contingent also made its point with dramatic visuals, including 200 large foamcore placards with silk-screened images on front and back. One side was a picture of a nightmarish barracks-style shelter rubber-stamped U.S. GOV'T APPROVES AIDS WARE-HOUSING; the other showed a typical city apartment block and urged HUMANE HOUSING FOR PEOPLE WITH AIDS.

Photo: Tom McKitterick

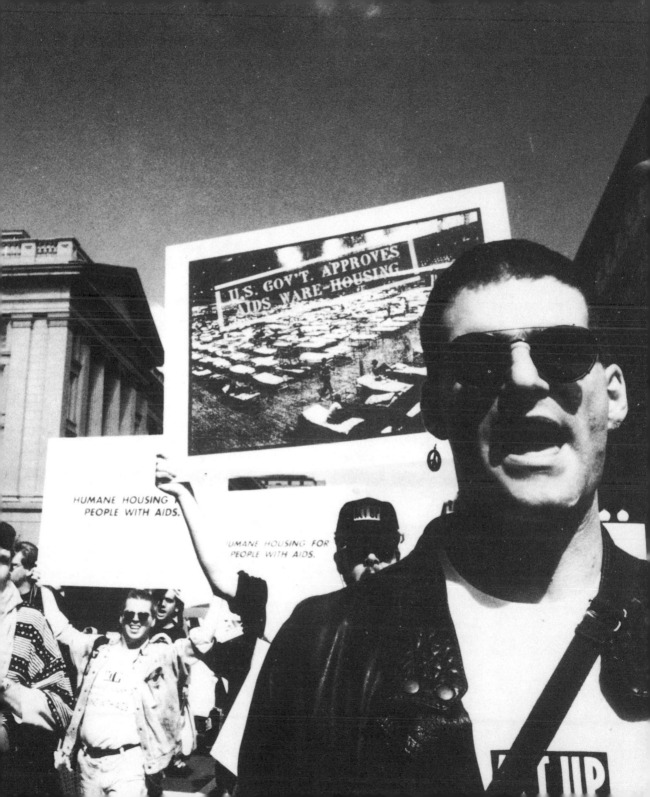

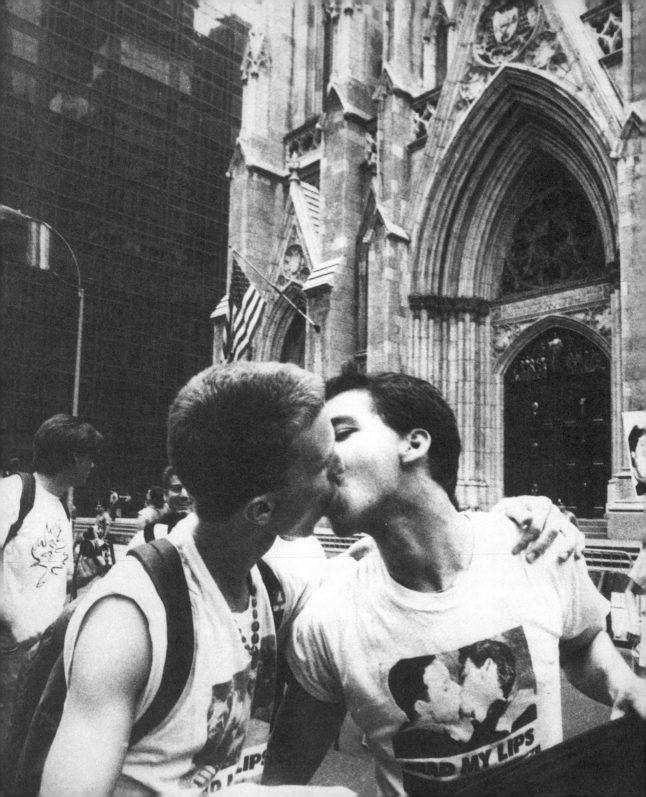

*St. Patrick's Cathedral, New York City,
December 10, 1989*

In 1987 the National Conference of Catholic Bishops agreed to allow a limited exception to the ban on contraceptives: because of the extraordinary circumstances of a dangerous epidemic, condom use as a protection against HIV infection would be minimally tolerated by the church. The archconservative Cardinal O'Connor of New York vehemently opposed the ruling and continued to rail against any kind of safe sex teaching other than abstinence within his jurisdiction. O'Connor had been made archbishop of New York in the spring of 1984 and appointed cardinal a year later by Pope John Paul II, whose conservative political and moral positions O'Connor could be counted on to enforce. From the moment he arrived in New York, O'Connor became an outspoken and powerful opponent of progressive politics, taking on the lesbian and gay movement as his particular obsession. The city's Gay Rights Bill was passed in 1986 over his fierce opposition, and he still refuses to abide by the antidiscrimination law in the provision of services contracted by the city. He banned masses held by the gay Catholic organization Dignity from Catholic churches and got an injunction to prevent the group's silent protests in St. Patrick's against the ban. The clear message from O'Connor's pulpit is that gay people are immoral, and fagbashers have taken heed: violence against lesbians and gays has sharply increased in the past decade.

But O'Connor's most directly murderous pronouncements have been about AIDS. He has consistently opposed safe sex education and the use of condoms to prevent HIV transmission. This would be lethal enough if it affected only obedient Catholics, but O'Connor's influence extends well beyond the docile minority. As soon as he came to New York he formed a close alliance with his fellow reactionary, Mayor Koch, whose policies were consistently informed by the cardinal's "moral" positions. This means, for one thing, that in the p u b l i c schools, where 85 percent of the students are people of color, AIDS education has been a just-say-no harangue–antigay, antisex, antilife. Statistics show that by the end of high school the vast majority of students are sexually active and many use drugs. Preaching abstinence denies their reality and will ultimately deny many of them their lives.

Photo: Ben Thornberry

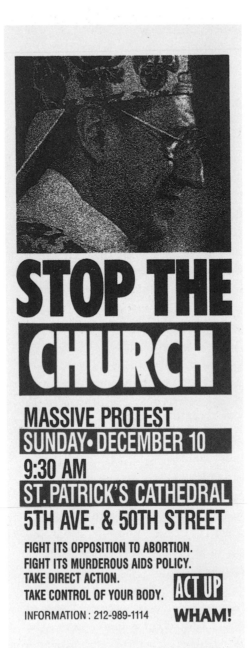

STOP THE CHURCH

MASSIVE PROTEST
SUNDAY • DECEMBER 10
9:30 AM
ST. PATRICK'S CATHEDRAL
5TH AVE. & 50TH STREET

FIGHT ITS OPPOSITION TO ABORTION.
FIGHT ITS MURDEROUS AIDS POLICY.
TAKE DIRECT ACTION.
TAKE CONTROL OF YOUR BODY.

INFORMATION : 212-989-1114

ACT UP
WHAM!

In early November 1989, the National Conference of Catholic Bishops, under pressure from O'Connor and his conservative cronies in the church hierarchy, rescinded the bishops' earlier stance on condom use to prevent HIV transmission. They now demand total abstinence as the only means of prevention, even if one partner in a sanctioned marriage is HIV-infected. A few weeks later, the Vatican held its first conference on AIDS, where the pope reaffirmed the church's condemnation of homosexuality and ban on all forms of contraception. Monsignor Carlo Caffarra stated the church's attitude about condoms bluntly: their use "is a true and proper anticoncep-tive act which is never licit under any circumstances or for any reasons." A speech by a theologian from Liechtenstein suggested that AIDS could indeed be seen as God's wrath against homosexuality, leading an American attending the conference to call it "three days of gay-bashing." O'Connor was one of the prime bashers, saying in his speech, "I believe the greatest damage done to persons with AIDS is done by those health care profes-sionals who refuse to confront the moral dimensions of sexual aberrations or drug abuse." And he went on to claim, "The truth is not in condoms or clean needles. These are lies–lies perpetuated often for political reasons on the part of public health officials." Because such utter disregard for truth and outbursts of hatred toward the suffering are unseemly in a Christian, O'Connor attempted to temper his statements by claiming that he had "sat with, listened to, emptied the bedpans of, and washed the sores of more than 1,100 persons with AIDS." What he meant was that in the hospitals and nursing home facilities the taxpayers pay him to manage through city contracts, he and his minions daily inflict the indignity of their archaic moralism on people dying from a disease he is helping to spread.

ACT UP's plan to STOP THE CHURCH was formulated during the final stages of the fall mayoralty campaign. Because former U.S. prosecutor Rudolph Giuliani, a Catholic, was running on the Republican ticket against Democrat David Dinkins, the church's stranglehold over city politics became an even more pressing issue, as it also concerned a woman's right to choose an abortion. Giuliani waffled on choice, as he waffled on every politically charged subject, but the cardinal didn't. He openly supported Operation Rescue terrorism against family planning clinics and urged the creation of a new order of nuns whose mission would be fighting abortion rights. ACT UP had been active in the struggle to keep abortion legal and accessible for some time by joining counterdemonstrations when

Stop the Church,
1989,
Vincent Gagliostro.
Crack-and-peel sticker,
offset lithography,
6½ × 2½".

Operation Rescue's well-financed intimidation squads attacked New York clinics. ACT UP's support of abortion rights was not solely a matter of individual members' political convictions or of our coalition-building with other progressive movements. Apart from the philosophical links between the AIDS activist and pro-choice positions on control of one's own body and health care rights, there are even more direct connections between AIDS and reproductive rights issues. Women are routinely excluded from AIDS drug trials because of their "reproductive capacities" (drug companies' concerns about endangering fetuses are, of course, really fears of potential law suits). Women are forced to accept sterilization to gain entry into some trials; and often HIV-positive pregnant women are coerced into having abortions against their will. The ACT UP Women's Committee had thoroughly documented these facts and presented them to the entire group within the context of a March 1989 teach-in on women and AIDS. Their WOMEN AND AIDS HANDBOOK of more than 100 pages became a primer on the subject, providing essential background information on the present status of women in the United States, the history of women and the medical establishment, and the relationship of the feminist health movement to the AIDS activist movement.

Know Your Scumbags,
1989,
Richard Deagle and
Victor Mendolia.
Subway advertising poster,
offset lithography,
22 × 21"
(also used as placard).

Several busloads of ACT UP members traveled to Washington, D.C., to form a contingent at the huge pro-choice demonstration there on April 9, 1989. We added our militant voices to those of NO MORE NICE GIRLS in an otherwise rather staid march, our chant proclaiming

ACT UP, WE'RE HERE.
WE'RE LOUD AND RUDE, PRO–CHOICE AND QUEER.

Three months later the conservative majority on the Supreme Court struck another severe blow to abortion rights in *Webster v. Reproductive Health Services.* Although the historic *Roe v. Wade* decision guaranteeing a woman's constitutional right to an abortion was not entirely overturned, the states were now given so much power to restrict access to abortions that in some states many women effectively no longer have the right to choose at all. This is the case in Missouri, where *Webster* was initiated and whose law bans abortion, including counseling and referral, from any institution receiving public funding (poor women have had no meaningful right to choose since the Hyde Amendment denied federal Medicaid payments for abortion).

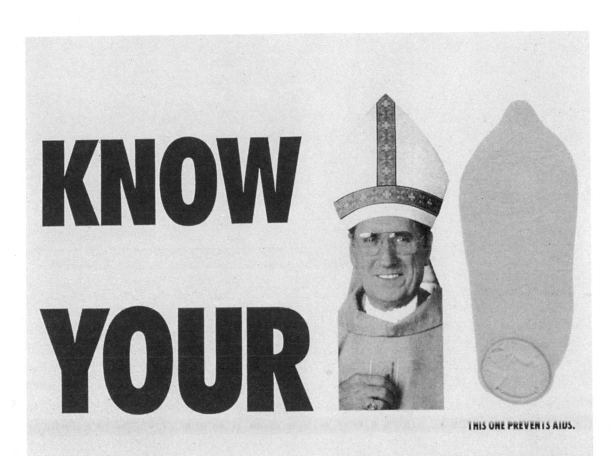

THIS ONE PREVENTS AIDS.

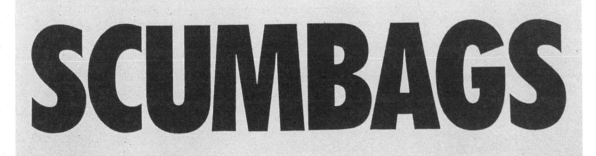

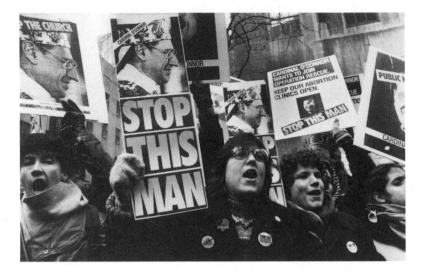

ACT UP and WHAM! demonstrators at St. Patrick's Cathedral, New York City, December 10, 1989 (photo: T. L. Litt).

In response to *Webster*, abortion rights forces reorganized and became more militant. The New York group WHAM! (Women's Health Action and Mobilization) staged a number of direct actions and teamed up with ACT UP to organize STOP THE CHURCH. Our demo scenario called for a legal picket around St. Patrick's, culminating in a mass "die-in," a tactic of playing dead in the streets often used by ACT UP to symbolize what the protest target was doing to us. At the same time, affinity groups secretly planned civil disobedience inside the cathedral while O'Connor said mass. More than 4,500 people showed up at St. Patrick's Sunday morning to STOP CHURCH INTERFERENCE IN OUR LIVES. Carrying signs saying STOP THIS MAN, CURB YOUR DOGMA, and DANGER, NARROW-MINDED CHURCH AHEAD, we loudly protested THE SEVEN DEADLY SINS OF CARDINAL O'CONNOR AND CHURCH POLITICIANS:

- ASSAULT ON LESBIANS AND GAYS. In the Ratzinger Letter on the pastoral "care of homosexuals," the church declares that people should not be surprised when a "morally offensive lifestyle is physically attacked." This position encourages the escalating violence against lesbians and gays.

- BIAS. Church-governed "morality" and public policy have been militantly opposed to the repeal of antilesbian and antigay discriminatory laws and criminal sodomy statutes. The cardinals and bishops cannot impose their rules on our bodies and our lives.

- IGNORANT DENIAL. In Rome, O'Connor addressed the Vatican Conference on AIDS, stating "good morality is good medicine." No form of church morality can comfort a homeless person with AIDS or get needed medical treatment to people who are sick.

- ENDANGERING WOMEN'S LIVES. O'Connor stated, "I wish I could join Operation Rescue," while urging all "good" Catholics to escalate their attacks on abortion rights and women's health facilities. The National Conference of Catholic Bishops chose O'Connor to spearhead the church's antiabortion political movement. O'Connor's response: "We have to be more aggressive. That's what my bones are telling me." To be "more aggressive," O'Connor proposes an order of nuns dedicated to full-time legal, medical, and political opposition to abortion.

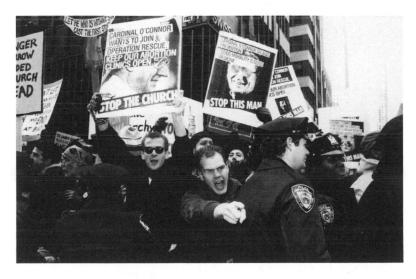

ACT UP and WHAM! demonstrators behind police barricades at St. Patrick's Cathedral, New York City, December 10, 1989 (photo: Ellen B. Neipris).

- NO SAFE SEX EDUCATION. O'Connor openly opposes education about sex, safer sex, contraception, condoms, and AIDS in both parochial and public schools. The archdiocese has also opposed safe sex education in AIDS health care facilities, even when these facilities have been donated by the city. By advocating abstinence as the only means of prevention, O'Connor denies reality, denies lifesaving information, and endangers all of our lives.

- NO CONDOMS. Opposition to condom use from the National Conference of Catholic Bishops and O'Connor is a major component in the continued spread of AIDS and is **k i l l i n g** people. HIV infection is now believed to be growing fastest among adolescents. Without immediate information about preventive methods, including condom use, people will continue to die.

- NO CLEAN NEEDLES. Sharing needles is the most frequent mode of transmission for new cases of HIV infection in New York City. The National Conference of Catholic Bishops opposes needle exchange programs, which supply clean needles to IV drug users, as a "quick fix solution." New York's drug treatment programs have a six-month waiting list; sterile syringes can protect a drug user from HIV infection.

During high mass inside the church, angry protestors forced O'Connor to abandon his sermon. Affinity groups lay down in the aisles, threw condoms in the air, chained themselves to pews, or shouted invectives at the cardinal. One former altar boy deliberately dropped a consecrated Communion wafer on the floor. (The media had a field day with that one: by the day after the event, it had become legions of sacrilegious "homosexual activists" desecrating the host.) Forty-three activists were arrested and dragged out of the cathedral; another 68 were arrested in the streets.

Media coverage was extensive, distorted, negative. The immensely powerful Cardinal O'Connor was portrayed as a helpless martyr. "All hatred is terribly disturbing," he was quoted as saying, as if it were not *his* hatred that was at issue. To the press, the politicians, and even to conservative gay "leaders," STOP THE CHURCH went too far: because we went inside the cathedral, we denied Catholic parishioners their freedom of religion. Their rights became the focus; our life-and-death issues were secondary.

Because ACT UP meetings are open to anyone who wants to come to the Lesbian and Gay Community Services Center, the police and others always know of our plans in advance. O'Connor was thus informed and perfectly prepared for our assault. He filled the church not with the usual Sunday faithful, but with Catholic militants and undercover police. Mayor Koch was also there to side with his old buddy. When the sermon was shouted down, O'Connor had photocopies of it ready to hand out. The heavily reported "outrage" of the parishioners at the disruption of the mass was therefore completely orchestrated. If that was to be expected, so too was the brutality of the New York City police, the majority of whom are Irish and Italian Catholics. The barricaded area for the legal picket was so tight as to make us feel like caged animals and incite us to violence, which *we*

Public Health Menace,

1989,

Vincent Gagliostro.

Poster, photocopy,

24 × 18"

(also used as placard).

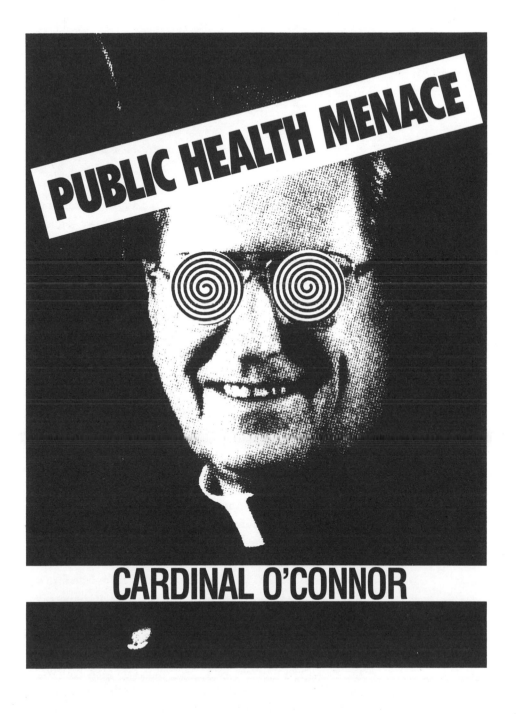

nevertheless resisted. Outside the barricades, though, one demonstrator was dragged into a doorway and kicked repeatedly in the groin by the good Christian cops. The press noticed none of this. They worried about that wafer.

It had been difficult to build consensus in ACT UP about STOP THE CHURCH. We knew the Catholic church would not change its positions, and we predicted that the media would misrepresent the target of the demonstration as Catholics or Catholicism, rather than the church hierarchy's impact on all of us through the power illegally granted them by the state. But follow-up debate declared STOP THE CHURCH a success on several counts. The demo sent out the message that there aren't any barriers we won't cross—with the exception of our pledge to nonviolence—in order to help save lives. It proved that we can build effective coalitions with other activist movements dedicated to the rights of health care and control over our own bodies. And it made us rededicate ourselves to protecting one another in the face of violence used against us.

Perhaps even more important, STOP THE CHURCH taught us the necessity of applying rigorous political analysis to our choice of targets, with the goal of productive change uppermost in our minds. As soon as STOP THE CHURCH was over, we began strategizing for the second decade of the AIDS epidemic. And in the first weeks of the 1990s, off we went—to Albany to disrupt Governor Mario Cuomo's state-of-the-state address with our demand that he recognize AIDS as a STATE OF EMERGENCY, an emergency in housing and social services, in health care, and in drug treatment. And to Atlanta, Georgia, to demand that the Centers for Disease Control broaden the definition of AIDS to include all HIV-related illnesses, especially those not now counted because they are specific to women.

Less than three weeks into the new decade, though, we learned the hard way just how little we can depend on, how much harder we have to fight. On January 19, 1990, Mayor David Dinkins, the man we'd helped elect, appointed Dr. Woodrow A. Myers, Jr., health commissioner of New York City. Formerly health commissioner of Indiana, Myers was one of that "batch of geeks and unknowns" appointed to Reagan's original Presidential Commission on the HIV Epidemic. In Indiana he supported mandatory name reporting, contact tracing, and quarantine. He failed to disburse grants from the Centers for Disease Control to AIDS organizations, and he opposed PWA representation on the state AIDS advisory council. ACT UP

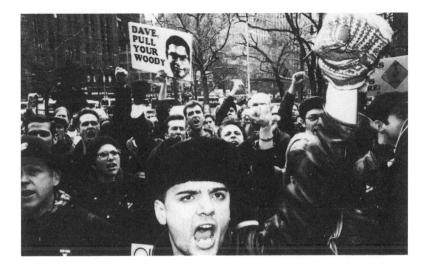

ACT UP demonstrators protest the appointment of Woodrow A. Myers, Jr., as New York City health commissioner, City Hall, New York City, January 19, 1990 (photo: Tom McKitterick).

worked tirelessly against the appointment, but we lost. The day the delayed appointment was finally made, the *New York Times* editorialized for Myers and against ACT UP. Deploying a standard deceit, the *Times* called us "a gay activist group" and pitted us against the interests of people of color (Myers is Black). The *Times*'s divisive tactic is consistently used against us. It pretends that *we* are all gay—and white, that there's no such thing as a gay person of color, and most insidiously, that opposing punitive AIDS policies that will endanger everyone is a selfish "homosexual" obsession. Castigating Dinkins for the little attention he did pay to ACT UP and our allies, the *Times* editorial ended, "To turn down Dr. Myers because of the hypothetical fears of a vocal minority would be an error."

But in spite of the betrayal represented by Myers's appointment, and in spite of the *New York Times*'s unceasing incomprehension of AIDS activists and the interests we promote, we also won a historic victory. For nearly a week, the New York news media focused on what they termed the first serious political crisis of David Dinkins's mayoralty—his dispute with ACT UP over who should direct city AIDS policy. During the press conference to announce the appointment, Dinkins was conciliatory toward ACT UP, insisting that "we have not come to a parting of the ways." Myers asked for a meeting with ACT UP. In less than three years, our movement has achieved enough recognition, enough respect, enough *power*, that the mayor of New York City cannot ignore us. Now we must teach him, and Woody Myers, that they owe us much more.

DOUGLAS CRIMP, recipient of the 1988 Frank Jewett Mather Award for distinction in art criticism, is the editor of *AIDS: Cultural Analysis/Cultural Activism*. ADAM ROLSTON is an architect and artist. Both are active members of ACT UP New York.